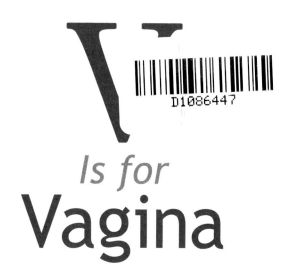

*Is for*

Vagina

# V

## *Is for*
# Vagina

Your **A**-to-**Z** Guide to
Periods, Piercings, Pleasures
*and so much more*

Alyssa Dweck, MS, MD, FACOG and Robin Westen

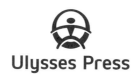

**Ulysses Press**

Published by: ULYSSES PRESS
P.O. Box 3440
Berkeley, CA 94703
www.ulyssespress.com

ISBN13: 978-1-61243-015-7
Library of Congress Control Number: 2011913378

Printed in the United States by Bang Printing

10 9 8 7 6 5 4 3 2 1

Acquisitions Editor: Kelly Reed
Managing Editor: Claire Chun
Editor: Paula Dragosh
Proofreader: Lauren Harrison
Indexer: Sayre Van Young
Cover design: Wade Nights
Cover illustration: © mtmmarek/fotolia.com
Illustration on page 10: © Evan K. Krakovitz MD
Production: Judith Metzener

Distributed by Publishers Group West

To Evan, my husband. You are my rock.
—*Alyssa Dweck, MD*

As always to my husband, Howie, my mentor, friend, and lover—and to sister goddesses everywhere.
—*Robin Westen*

# Contents

## Your V, A to Z

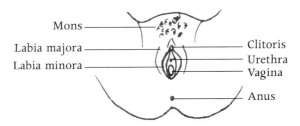

# Introduction

Vaginas. I've seen *thousands* of them. As a full-time practicing OB/GYN for almost two decades, I've learned women have a complex relationship with their V's. Whether curious, closed, excited, elated, tenacious, mortified, tearful, or fearful, shy, panicked, pugnacious, even petrified, women first and foremost all want to know one thing: *Am I normal down there?*

This essential question is the reason that I'm Facebooked frequently, cornered in the grocery store aisle, sidelined at the gym, questioned in cafés, and stopped on the street by women who have urgent issues about their vaginas. Their queries and concerns inspired me to write *V Is for Vagina*. Rather than talk yeast infection in the produce aisle or labioplasty on the elliptical machine, I wanted to get the word out, to educate women in an easy-to-read, nonthreatening, down-to-earth way. I wanted to share medically sound and up-to-date information in a humorous, hip, and relaxed style. And I wanted to have a little fun, too.

So, here it is, *V Is for Vagina*: a humorous but informative guide to the sometimes mysterious but always fascinating and amazing VAGINA. Some of the chapters ahead are more "medical," while others are chatty and lighthearted. There's material that may embarrass some readers, even offend others. But please be assured that all of the information is solid and stems from the experiences I've been fortunate enough to share with my patients over the years. Nothing, and I mean *nothing*, surprises me anymore. Truly, I've heard it all.

You can either use *V Is for Vagina* as a reference guide to answer your individual questions or take the quiz at the beginning of the book to figure out where you stand in general V knowledge. From there, you can fill in the blanks by reading those sections that need clarification. It's also a great companion to take along for a women's day out with your BFFs. I only suggest you keep your voices down if you're in public. Even uttering the word *vagina* can quickly draw the attention of strangers! And moms, this guide can help you explain the basics to your young daughters in a heart-centered and nonscary way.

> This to my mind is the vagina as icon,
> Sacred, inviolable, worshipped.
> The sister and source
> From which all human life springs.
> —*Catherine Blackledge*

But of course, never substitute the information in this book for a visit with your gynecologist if you still have questions—or need medical attention.

Ready for the inside scoop on your lovely V?

Please read, laugh, and learn ...

# Let's Have a Party: The Vagina Is Coming Out!

Just as women's bodies are softer than men's, so their understanding is sharper.

—*Christine de Pisan*

*OUR V*: It's the subject of girl talk over coffee, blabbed about on *Grey's Anatomy*, discussed by Oprah, described on *Curb Your Enthusiasm*, joked over on *Bill Maher*, rapped on by Lil Wayne, mocked in *Date Night*, enjoyed on *Sex and the City,* painted on canvas, represented in caves, sculpted into walls, monologued on Broadway, banned, beautified, deified, pierced, waxed, creamed, oiled, stretched, tightened, tattooed, glorified, despised, and mythologized. There are over one thousand slang words for it (*who-ha, vajayjay, cha-cha, lady flower, foo foo, cooch, noonie, love clam, twinkle, quim, the love canal, the great gorge, pink, pussy, salmon canyon,* and *oasis,* to name just a few). You can order mugs, T-shirts, songs, poems, pens, pencils, sculptures, paintings, posters, and magnets with the word *vagina* in, over, or on them.

And suddenly there seems to be a market for putting the va-va-voom back in the vajayjay. The number of women undergoing cosmetic surgery to improve its function and appearance—tighten the V, sculpt the labia, or restore the hymen—has gone up dramatically in the last few years, making thcm procedure the fastest growing in the country. Spas in New York, L.A., D.C., and elsewhere offer "vagina rejuvenation," everything from irrigating the vaginal passage, slipping in a "breath" mint, or massaging the clit to boost its sensitivity, to applying a tightening cream that promises to reduce its appearance to a "youthful" state for a full twenty-four hours. Think Cinderella having a ball!

Yet, despite all the attention, most of us know squat about our salmon canyon. For example, Summer's Eve, a women's hygiene product, recently surveyed sisters from all backgrounds across the United States and found that nearly 70 percent of women asked cannot identify five major parts of their female genitalia, and nearly 60 percent struggle with unresolved feelings just about the word *vagina*.

Need more evidence that when it comes to our lovely V's we're in the dark but want and *need* to be brought into the light? Consider these stats from the Association of Reproductive Professionals:

- While women perform breast self-exams regularly, only half (49%) surveyed have *ever* performed a self-exam of their vaginas. Twenty-four percent have not looked at their vagina in a year or longer. HOW SAD.
- Two-thirds of women (65%) concur that vaginal health and research have not received the proper attention they deserve. AGREED.

- More than half of the women surveyed (59%) say that society has too many misconceptions about vaginas. TOTALLY.
- Ninety percent of women agree that it's important for women to be sufficiently educated about the vagina. *HELLO* … THAT'S WHY I'M HERE.
- Nearly three in four women surveyed (73%) believe that the vagina is still a shocking topic. GULP.
- Some women consider their vaginas "ugly," "gross," "dirty," and "embarrassing." LET ME SAY THIS RIGHT NOW—*THIS HAS GOT TO STOP!*
- Only half of the women surveyed (51%) consider themselves to be extremely/very knowledgeable about their vaginas. LET'S CHANGE THAT!

The good news is this: Times are changing, *fast* and *furiously*. After all, just in the past few years, women have had to deal with plenty of new and different issues, including infections from the oh-so-popular and bare-it-all Brazilian wax, piercings gone awry, tattoos run amok, and irritation from speed-breaking spinning classes. There are updates on estrogen replacement; a controversial vaccine to protect young girls from getting genital warts and cervical cancer; the redesign of tampons and pads; a host of new and ultratitillating sex toys; the current vajazzling craze; updated consideration on vitamins and soy; new treatments for vulvodynia, the vaginal pain syndrome thousands of women suffer; and OMG, so much more. Plus, sex researchers have discovered the "A spot," which some claim one-ups the "G spot" for guaranteeing over-the-top orgasm pleasure.

> For women the best aphrodisiacs are words. The G spot is in the ears. He who looks for it below there is wasting his time.
> —*Isabel Allende*

Yes, women crave the inside scoop on their quims. Maybe that's why Google has over 21 million entries for *vagina*. We want to be in on the latest *everything* about *everything*, from self-exams, tampons, Pap tests, cunnilingus, allergies, birth, yeast infections, and semen allergies to ingrown pubic hairs, Kegels, lubricants, and more... *much* more.

But first things first: Let's take a look through the cultural kaleidoscope, because the vagina deserves a historical view. After all, everybody begins with the vagina in some way: You were conceived and born, right? Or as Catherine Blackledge, author of the comprehensive *The Story of V*, writes: "The vagina is the seat of female sexual pleasure, the site of the creation of humankind and the channel for its birth."

The self-proclaimed feminist author Naomi Wolf sees our cha-cha from a historical perspective:

> The way we understand and envision the vagina at certain moments in history is a metaphor for how we are willing to see women in general and how women are encouraged to see themselves. From the Greeks and the Romans to Freud, from pornography and health to goddesses, from worship to denigration and even mutilation, there is a history of this wonderful organ, the "dark continent" of female sexuality, well deserving of its own story.

True, the historical, artistic, and literary record of our who-has is awesome, mirroring our culture's view of sexuality. Before the nineteenth century, terms for the

V were affectionate and kind. Even the word *cunt,* one of the oldest words for female genitalia, was intended to mean something warm and cuddly. In fact, before the fifteenth century, *cunt* was just another word, so much a part of everyday vocabulary that it was used in naming public streets. Around 1230, for example, there was a London street called *Gropecuntelane,* and in Paris there was a *Rue Grateecon,* which translates as "Scratchcunt Street." But after the fifteenth century, *cunt* was totally taboo. In England it was forbidden in speech and print, and it was a legal offense to publish the word.

But get this: The much tamer word, *vagina,* is *still* illegal to use in the United States in commercials, even when the product being hawked is a tampon! Thank goodness this uptight, V-dissing perspective isn't the whole story. In fact, throughout history, cultures all over the world have at times celebrated the gorgeous, glorious lady flower. Vagina art can be found in archaic statuettes, amulets, and figurines, as well as carved on seals and jewelry, and in sculptures, installations, and paintings in our modern museums.

Way back in the Paleolithic era, images of vulvas were painted or carved and emblazoned on various Stone Age sites in France, Spain, Russia, and other locations. Perhaps one of the most striking views of the V can be seen on the walls of a cave in Vienne, France. Here a trinity of vulvas was carved on the rock surface as far back as seventeen thousand years ago!

Then in 1896 German archaeologists discovered a temple site in Turkey dating back to the fifth century BCE, and within it were seven petite terra-cotta females. What makes them so fantabulous is the artist created these little sculptures so that the face, stomach, and genitals merge into one image. Indeed they are, without dispute, total vulva women.

But these little gals won't take the proverbial Honey Pot Award for most outstanding vulva. That may go to a figurine dating back to between twenty-one thousand and twenty-three thousand years ago, carved out of limonite and found in southern France. This Venus figurine displays a huge, curved oval vulva that's slit right down the center.

Some of the oldest examples of skirt-lifting and vulva-revealing images date from fourteen thousand years ago and are found on a Syrian cylinder seal. One can easily see three women either spreading their legs wide or lifting their clothes to reveal with pride and without prejudice their impressive V's.

Historians say it's amazing that these kinds of vulvanic works of art survive, considering that by the seventeenth century so many were ordered hidden, destroyed, buried, or burned.

African culture was slow to condemn V exposure. As recently as the twentieth century, a common shaming gesture in plenty of African societies was exposing the vulva, as if to say "Hey, don't forget where you came from, buddy."

In other parts of the world, vulvas created by natural rock formations are still venerated. For instance, in Japan, parents encourage their children to play near rocks that resemble genitals. Especially renowned is a group of formations in Kyushu. It's believed these shapes offer good luck and health to anyone within their vicinity. Same goes in Thailand on the island of Koah Samui. Two natural vulva rock formations in the cliffs overlooking the sea are used as a place not only of prayer but of pilgrimage as well. Tourists who visit the sexy formations in the morning hours will see native Thais leaving flower offerings on the sacred spot.

*The Sanskrit word for vagina is yoni, meaning womb, origin, source, and universe.*

And let's not forget the V-loving ancient Egyptians. They focused on the downward-pointing triangle shape and made it the symbol of sacred creativity. Perhaps that's why the entrance to the queen's chamber in the pyramid of Cheops is indicated by a downward-pointing triangle. BTW: If you could exam it, the same triangle is seen in the interior structure of the uterus. And, not to be left out, Tantric lore also expresses the vagina as the entrance to the past as well as the future.

Speaking of interior views, the famous Taoist text "The Wondrous Discourse of Su Nu" explains how vaginas come in eight varieties and sizes. From smallest to largest, they are known as:

- The Zither or Lute String
- The Water-caltrop Teeth or Water-chestnut Teeth
- The Peaceful Valley or Little Stream
- The Dark or Mysterious Pearl
- The Valley Seed or Valley Proper
- The Palace of Delight or Deep Chamber
- The Inner Door or Gate of Prosperity
- The North Pole

Reiner de Graaf, who was a brilliant sixteenth-century Dutch physician, anatomist, and admirer of the V, made major discoveries in reproductive biology. He was effusive and poetic about the vagina's ability to be the perfect hostess. Get this:

> The woman's vagina is so cleverly constructed that it will accommodate itself to each and every penis; it will go out to meet a short one, retire before a long one, dilate for a fat one, and constrict for a thin one. Nature has taken account every variety of penis, and so there is no need solicitously to seek a scabbard the same size as your knife…. Every man can thus come together with every woman and every woman with every man.

With this understanding in mind, it's not surprising vibrators took off at home as well as in the doc's office. Even in the uptight United States, as early as the 1890s, women could purchase a $5 portable vibrator advertised as "perfect for weekend trips" instead of paying their doctor $2 a visit to stimulate the clitoris until reaching orgasm. Hmmm … not sure if that would be covered under insurance today.

But there's no doubt the vagina is versatile. Today extraordinary muscle control can be witnessed mostly during sex industry shows. Smoking cigarettes, firing Ping-Pong balls, writing messages, opening bottles, and picking up sushi with chopsticks are just a few of the many tricks of the trade.

Sadly though, in some cultures, there's no celebration of the V's versatility and ability to feel pleasure. Whether it's called female genital cutting, female circumcision, female genital mutilation, or cliterectomy, it's a surgical procedure ranging from drawing blood to removing the clitoris by itself, to removing the external genitals, joining the sides, and leaving a small opening. This horrendous practice dates to ancient times; usually performed on young girls and in a ritual context, it's purported by its practitioners to guard a girl's virginity and reduce her sexual desires. Because it's usually undertaken in unhygienic conditions, even today, cutting may lead to severe bleeding, infection, debilitating pain, and death. The long-term consequences of this barbaric practice can include an inability to urinate or expel menstrual blood, pain during sexual intercourse, and prolonged childbirth.

Let's Get Sentimental: The Romans borrowed Eros from the Greeks and named him Cupid. Eros has been depicted in art in many ways. The Romans regarded him as a symbol of life after death, and the Greeks put him everywhere from drinking vessels to oil flasks, usually showing him ready to fire an arrow into the heart of an unsuspecting "victim."

Rather than end this section on a sad note, let's celebrate our amazing cha-cha with modern literary and art works. This book would not be complete without giving kudos to Eve Ensler, author of the iconic work *The Vagina Monologues*. Ensler, who brought the vagina right out of the genital closet, interviews a diverse group of over two hundred women about their vaginas: young and old; married and single; heterosexual, bisexual, and lesbian; working-class women, professional women, and sex workers; women of various ethnicities. As the author points out, some of the monologues are verbatim, some are composites, and some are her invented impressions. The subjects, which all have to do with vaginas, include such topics as what a vagina looks like, what goes in and comes out of vaginas, menstruation and birth, and more playfully, "If your vagina got dressed, what would it wear?" or "If your vagina could talk, what would it say, in two words?"

Breaking the vagina visual art barrier was the feminist artist Judy Chicago with her groundbreaking work *The Dinner Party*, an installation of ceramic vagina place settings representing thirty-nine mythical and historical famous women, produced from 1974 to 1979. Despite art-world resistance to her vagina theme, it toured sixteen venues in six countries on three continents to a viewing audience of 1 million. Since 2007 it's been on permanent exhibition at the Brooklyn Museum in New York City.

More recently, there's the quim work by Jamie McCartney, an artist from Brighton, UK. McCartney convinced over four hundred women, ages ranging from eighteen to seventy-six, to spread their legs so he could make a plaster cast of their vaginas and vulvas and display them en masse. McCartney's socially conscious installation was five years in the making. Included in his piece are mothers and daughters, identical twins, transgendered men and women, as well as a woman pre- and postnatal and another pre- and postlabioplasty. McCartney's work uses shock, humor, and spectacle—ultimately educating people about what normal women *really* look like.

Hallelujah!

# How Much Do You Know About Your V?

## Test Your V Knowledge

1. *How many women won't have an orgasm with intercourse alone?*
   a. 10 percent
   b. 50 percent
   c. 75 percent

2. *Who discovered the G spot?*
   a. Walt Disney. It's make-believe.
   b. Helen Gurley Brown, iconic editor of *Cosmopolitan* magazine.
   c. Ernst Grafenberg, a German gynecologist.

3. *Why is it okay to have sex during pregnancy?*
   a. You wouldn't be horny if it weren't.
   b. The baby is protected within the uterus, cushioned by fluid.
   c. It's not! Abstain!

4. *The morning-after pill is:*
   a. A modern contraceptive method.
   b. A treatment to prevent pregnancy after unprotected sex.
   c. Only a dream.

5. *Yeast infections can be caused by:*
   a. Wearing panty liners.
   b. Taking antibiotics.
   c. Both of the above.

6. *What can you do if you believe your labia are too "fat"?*
   a. Consider (carefully) labioplasty.
   b. Do special labia exercises.
   c. Go on a diet and you'll lose weight down there, too.

7. *What is the "Transition Zone"?*
   a. The end of fertility and the start of menopause.
   b. An area of the cervix where squamous and glandular cells meet.
   c. A one-way ticket to incredible orgasms.

8. *Who* doesn't *need a Pap smear?*
   a. Women who are younger than sixteen and have not had sexual intercourse.
   b. Most women between the ages of thirty and forty.
   c. Women who have had a hysterectomy and kept their cervix.

9. *What are vulvar skin tags?*
   a. A potential sign of cancer. See your doctor immediately.
   b. Outgrowths of normal skin. No worries.
   c. Smooth white bumps under the surface of your vulva's skin.

10. *What's a common cause of low sex drive?*
    a. Sugar
    b. Exercise
    c. Poor body image

11. *What helps reduce the pain after a bikini wax?*
    a. Don't tan down there for twenty-four hours before and after the procedure.
    b. Wearing Spanx.
    c. Getting weekly waxes.

12. *What's the most popular place to pierce the vagina?*
    a. Inner labia
    b. Clitoral hood
    c. Outer labia

13. *Who made "vajazzling" famous?*
    a. Carrie Bradshaw
    b. Jennifer Love Hewitt
    c. Lady Gaga

14. *To keep your lady flower lovely:*
    a. Douche frequently.
    b. Take bubble baths.
    c. Wear cotton underwear (or go commando).

15. *Can women get addicted to porn?*
    a. No way!
    b. Yes! Duh.
    c. Porn addiction in women is rare.

16. *Both gonorrhea and chlamydia are treated with:*
    a. Antibiotics
    b. Douching
    c. Abstinence

17. *What can relieve menstrual cramps?*
    a. Chocolate
    b. Sex
    c. Aerobics

18. *Many women going through menopause experience:*
    a. Hot flashes
    b. Cramps
    c. Weight loss

19. *A woman trying to get pregnant should have intercourse:*
    a. On days one to four of a twenty-eight-day cycle.
    b. Only on day fourteen of a twenty-eight-day cycle.
    c. Depending on your cycle length, around ovulation, approximately days ten to nineteen.

20. *Tampons have been linked to which of the following diseases:*
    a. HIV
    b. Toxic shock syndrome
    c. Cervical cancer

21. *What is a leading cause of infertility?*
    a. Sexually transmitted diseases
    b. Psychological problems
    c. Lack of physical activity

22. *If you notice a pinpoint hole in your diaphragm you should:*
    a. Plug it up with contraceptive gel.
    b. Get a new diaphragm.
    c. Do nothing; it's unlikely that sperm will get through.

23. *During perimenopause, you should continue using some sort of contraception:*
    a. Until you skip a period.
    b. Until it's been a full year without your period.
    c. You don't need birth control during perimenopause.

24. *The following is true about HPV:*
    a. You're fully protected from transmission by using a condom.
    b. It's an uncommon virus, and even if you've had only two or three sex partners in your lifetime, you're unlikely to get it.
    c. In most instances, HPV will not lead to cervical cancer.

25. *A colposcopy is:*
    a. A form of birth control.
    b. A microscopic exam of the cervix to check for abnormal cells.
    c. A new gynecological app for your iPhone.

26. *A Bartholin's cyst can be treated in all of the following ways except:*
    a. Warm soaks, pain medication, and drainage.
    b. Leaving it alone; it may go away by itself.
    c. Having a lot of sex so it'll pop.

27. *You can prevent a urinary tract infection by all the following except:*
    a. Wiping from front to back after going to the bathroom.
    b. Holding in your urine all day.
    c. Urinating before and after sex.

28. True or False: *Vaginal discharge is always a yeast infection.*

29. True or False: *Low libido has one cause, low hormone levels, and a simple pill will cure it.*

30. True or False: *Bleeding from the rectum is always due to hemorrhoids; evaluation is really not needed.*

31. True or False: *You can get genital herpes from oral sex.*

32. True or False: *The birth control pill offers protection against ovarian and uterine cancers.*

# Your V Score

Give yourself five points for each correct answer. Then total the score and read the analysis below to find out how much you really know about all things V!

| | | | |
|---|---|---|---|
| 1. C | 9. B | 17. B | 25. B |
| 2. C | 10. C | 18. A | 26. A |
| 3. B | 11. A | 19. C | 27. B |
| 4. B | 12. B | 20. B | 28. F |
| 5. C | 13. B | 21. A | 29. F |
| 6. A | 14. C | 22. B | 30. F |
| 7. B | 15. B | 23. B | 31. T |
| 8. A | 16. A | 24. C | 32. T |

## If You Scored between 140 and 160 Points

Congratulations, sister! You have above-average knowledge about your V as well as other areas of your femme health. This will not only serve your physical, emotional, and sexual needs but probably make you the go-to confidante to all your girlfriends who are feeling a little unsure about their lady flowers. But hold that bouquet! Sometimes being a know-it-all keeps women away from appointments they *should* make, especially an annual examination with the gynecologist. A smart, well-read, and savvy woman like you should remember to seek help when a problem arises. It's the perfect way to put your V knowledge to good use.

## If You Scored between 90 and 135 Points

You have a basic V knowledge, and that's one reason why you take such good care of your cha-cha and your other feminine health needs. But there are certain areas that can use a little more know-how. Go over your answers and find out where your smarts are shortchanged. Then look through the book to fill in the blanks and to get a better picture of what's going on down there. You've got potential to really grasp not only the fundamentals but also the finer points of female health. If you still have questions, don't be shy. Talk it over with your gynecologist and keep going until you get a deeper understanding. It's your body, after all.

## If You Scored *under* 85 Points

For you, it's pretty much a mystery down there. But if it helps you feel better about your low score, realize you're not alone. Lots of women are in the dark when it comes to their vaginas, and that's really a pity because it's such a fantastic part of you. You might have been brought up to feel shy or ashamed about your vag; it wasn't something discussed in your home or among your girlfriends. Even when you go to the doctor, you remain in the dark and never ask questions. Well! It's time to change all that. Turn the pages and read on. You'll not only learn what's going on in the land of your V, but you might be able to leave self-consciousness behind ... or at least take a few steps in that direction. Or as Miranda of *Sex and the City* so wisely put it: What's the big mystery?

# *Your V,*
# *A to Z*

The first lesson most of us learn as little girls is our ABCs, but it's not so simple when it comes to knowledge about our vaginas! Sometimes it takes research to dig down and find the facts. We thought using the familiar alphabet was the easiest, fastest, most familiar way for inquisitive women to locate the information they need and want about their V's. So whether you read the book in order from A to Z or just linger on a letter, you'll find what you're looking for—and probably lots more.

# A

# The A and G Spots and Every Erogenous Zone You've Ever Imagined! Plus O's and More O's!

Isn't it enough we're supposed to be the most awesome girlfriends, amazing moms, devoted wives, career-climbing professionals, and creative house organizers—now we're supposed to be XXX porn stars? Hey, only if you *want* to be! That said, here's the thing, girlfriend, you want to have a good (hey, make that *hot*, *sexy*, *transcendental*) time in bed. Otherwise, well, you might not only get bored right out of the bedroom, you could end up resenting your partner. And no one wants that. So let's get down and dirty, cover the basics, and then rev up your erogenous zones.

Sex is a beauty treatment! Scientific tests find that when women make love they produce amounts of the hormone estrogen, which makes hair shine and skin smooth.

# What Exactly Is an Orgasm?

Let's put it this way: When you're having one you probably won't hear the dryer buzzing, the dog whimpering to go out, your neighbors arguing, or *True Blood* in the background. But let's start with foreplay, where the most satisfying lovemaking sessions begin. That warm, *all is well with the world* feeling you're hopefully experiencing during foreplay is the rush of blood moving straight to your vajayjay and clit. Without getting *too* techie (and ruining the mood), it's around this time that the walls of your vagina start to secrete beads of lubrication that eventually get bigger and bigger and flow together. If that doesn't happen easily—no problemo: *Hello, helpful lube.*

About 75 percent of all women never reach orgasm from intercourse alone—that is, without the extra help of sex toys, hands, or tongue. And 10 to 15 percent never climax under any circumstances.

Onward: As you get hotter, blood continues to flood your pelvic area, and your breathing speeds up, heart rate increases, nipples get erect, and the lower part of your V narrows so it can grip the penis (if that's what's in there, or it could be a finger, dildo, or vibrator; or tongue, anyone?). If all goes swimmingly, a lovely amount of nerve and muscle tension builds up in your genitals, pelvis, buttocks, and thighs—until *yippee*—your body involuntarily releases all at once in a series of intensely pleasurable waves. Voilà! Your orgasm! Oh, girlfriend, if only life were *always* so easy breezy.

# I'm Almost There, about to Peak, and Then I Lose Momentum. What's Going On?

Nine times out of ten it's because you're probably not getting enough clitoral stimulation. You'll get close to orgasm, and your partner (or you, if you're masturbating) changes what he or she is doing. Or it could all be in your head. The fact is, for women, the largest erogenous zone is her brain. I mean, if you're thinking it's not going to happen or you're wondering whether those Prada shoes are still on sale, you might as well kiss the O good-bye.

About 1 percent of women can orgasm solely through breast stimulation. If you're one of them, lucky lady!

## True Or False? There's More Than Just One Erogenous Zone.

Oh, so very true! An erogenous zone is any area of your body that has heightened sensitivity, and the stimulation of it results in the production of sexual thrills! Women (and guys, too) have erogenous zones all over their bodies. But what turns one gal on may be a total turn-off to another. Sort of like ice cream flavors. Clit, eyelids, eyebrows, temples, shoulders, hands, arms, feet, hair, lips, neck, nipples, breasts, navel, thighs, wrists, behind the knees, hands … shall we go on? No, let your partner go on.

## What's This about the G Spot?

If you're asking, it probably means it hasn't been found—
*yet*! So let me get down to a little background and then the instructions. The G spot (some folks call it the urethral sponge) is wrapped around your urethra. When you're getting hot and bothered, the G spot swells with fluid and the juices push into your vagina where it's felt on the V wall. And, honey, it totally feels great! The best way to stimulate the G spot is through rhythmic massage with fingers, a penis, or dildo. It may take your partner practice

The G spot (or the Grafenberg spot) was named after the gynecologist Ernst Grafenberg in 1944.

to locate it. Plus, it might take some practice for you to connect with your G spot and learn how to experience the vaginal orgasms (which aren't nearly as common as clit orgasms) that are accompanied by its stimulation. But oooh—it's *so* worth it.

## So, Can I Find the G Spot Myself?

Sure, it's not hard to find at all. Just insert your index or middle finger into your vagina with your palm facing upward. You might have to use your middle finger if your G spot is located farther up the front wall. Once your finger is inside, make a "come here" motion with it—and that should pretty much do it.

## Whenever I Have a G Spot Orgasm It Feels Like I'm Peeing.

Oh, dear sister, not so. You've probably ejaculated. Beverley Whipple, an American sex guru and coauthor of the original G spot book, says that a vaginal orgasm may produce ejaculate—almost half a coffee cupful. It's true that some women leak a little urine during sex. But when urine leaks during sex, it's often during foreplay or vigorous intercourse, rather than during orgasm.

Q. What's the difference between a golf ball and a G spot?
A. A guy will spend two hours searching for a golf ball.

## What Is the A Spot?

The A spot is the anterior fornix, a spot on the front wall of the vagina—a few inches past the G spot that's rumored to induce orgasm. For your partner to reach it, you'll need to have your hips propped up on a pillow, move into missionary position, and have thrusts aimed high. Credibility Alert: Some folks say the A spot is a whole lotta hooey.

# B
## Oooh Baby, Baby

Giving birth is like taking your lower lip and forcing it over your head.

—*Carol Burnett*

If you've ever doubted for one itsy-bitsy second whether your vajayjay was truly wondrous, now that you've given birth you know what a silly girl you've been to even question it. Amazing, right? Yes, but also complicated. So let's get a good look at what's been happening lately to your lovely hothouse flower. And while we're at it, we'll also see why your sex drive may be on a chilly hiatus.

## Can I Have Sex When I'm Pregnant?

You're not alone if you're worrying about whether it's safe to have sexual intercourse during pregnancy. Unless your doctor has nixed the idea, you can have sex throughout the entire nine months. Whether you really want to is another story. And if you don't feel like it, sweetie, don't. There may be times when having sex is physically uncomfortable. Or you can experiment to find which positions are easiest. In general, during later pregnancy, you should avoid being flat on your back. Just know this: Sex is not harmful. Your baby is protected within the uterus and is cushioned by fluid. Of course, there are plenty of other ways to be intimate with your partner: cuddling, kissing, and fondling, mutual masturbation, and oral sex.

Bummer Alert: In certain circumstances, your doctor may advise against intercourse or orgasm during pregnancy.

## Sex *After* Birth or Is Someone Kidding Me?

*H-e-l-l-o libido, are you home?* It's only a few weeks post-delivery, and everything near the V zone (or higher up if you've had a C-section) could still be mighty sore. Even if you have a sex drive (ha ha), you're exhausted. As soon as you hit the bed, all you want to do is snore—oh, I mean sleep.

A recent study found that new moms who are over thirty-four or have had C-sections can reduce their risk of dangerous blood clots by avoiding hormonal birth control in the first forty-two days postpartum. *Isn't being postpartum its own form of birth control?*

Kidding aside, it's best to wait at least four to six weeks after delivery before having sex to allow time for your cervix to close, postpartum bleeding to stop, and any tears or repaired lacerations to heal. I know, just hearing this is sooooo sexy. And that doesn't even account for postpartum blues, changes in body image, and other obstacles. For instance, suddenly your number-one love object is your amazing baby.

Amy Corbin, blogger for Alphamom.com, wrote this about the six-week, no-sex window:

> While technically my gyno's instructions were simply "nothing in the vagina for six weeks," I chose to interpret it more as "DO NOT TOUCH ME, AT ALL. DO NOT EVEN THINK ABOUT TOUCHING ME. STOP LOOKING AT ME LIKE THAT." I was so horrified by the state of my body ... I just couldn't bear the thought of the squishing slapping awkwardness of sex when I didn't recognize the body I now had. What if my boobs leak? What if my stomach dangles?

It's not just new moms—some new dads are wary, too, about getting back in the saddle. I've had husbands actually come into my office at the six-week postpartum visit to hear it for themselves that sex is really okay now. The truth is, the chances of a problem occurring, like bleeding or infection, are small for about two weeks after giving birth. If you've had an episiotomy or a tear during birth, the site may be sore for a few weeks, and you probably should hold off on intercourse until it heals. Once and *if* you feel ready to have sex again, and your doctor has given you the go-ahead, it's a good idea to use a water-based lubricant and plenty of it. The vagina may be less moist than usual, especially if you're breast-feeding.

Even you're not having a period or are breast-feeding, you can become pregnant. Getting pregnant less than six months after giving birth can increase the risk of certain pregnancy problems, such as preterm birth. You should use some type of birth control when you start having sex again.

# My V Is Dripping

Well, honey pot, by now you probably know the quantity and quality of vaginal discharge in healthy women varies both individually and during your menstrual cycle. Slight odor and mild irritation can be normal. While pregnant, you'll also experience vaginal discharge (called leucor-rhea), which will be mucuslike, white or clear, without any other signs and symptoms such as itching, pain, burning or irritation, redness, or bleeding. If you're afraid you're trickling amniotic fluid or have an infection, don't hesitate to see your gyno.

# OMG! What Are These Bumps?

I'm frequently called by frantic pregnant patients describing a "cluster of grapes" bulging from their vulva. (Why is it always fruit? We'll discuss that philosophical question

### How to Deal with Varicose Veins

Sadly, you can't prevent varicose veins. But there are ways to help relieve swelling and soreness, and they may stop varicose veins from getting worse:

- If you must sit or stand for long periods, be sure to move around from time to time.

- Do not sit with your legs crossed.

- Prop up your legs—on your desk, a couch, a chair, or a footstool—as often as you can.

- Exercise—walk, swim, or ride an exercise bike.

- Wear support hose.

another time.) More often than not, these are varicose veins of the vulva; in medical terms, they're known as vulvar varicose veins. Here's what's going on: Now that you're pregnant, the weight of your uterus is pressing down on a major vein, which can slow blood flow from your lower body. The result may be sore, itchy, blue bulges on your legs and vulva.

Vulvar varicose veins are akin to hemorrhoids (bulging veins in the rectum). In most cases, it may seem gross, but varicose veins are not a problem. They usually improve or disappear after delivery.

## My Gyno Said I Had an Episiotomy. What *Exactly* Is It?

An episiotomy is pretty common, although it's not as routine a procedure as it used to be. The reason for an episiotomy—a cut made by a medical expert to your perineum, the space between your vagina and rectum—is to make delivery easier. Think open wider. There are a few options in the procedure. One is called a midline, or median, episiotomy. Doctors will tell you this type is easiest to perform, repair, and recover from. And with this approach, postpartum pain and discomfort during sex is less. The drawback is that there's a higher chance of a tear in the rectum or anal sphincter, which can lead to infection and future incontinence. A slightly different episiotomy procedure, called a mediolateral, minimizes the chance of sphincter or rectal involvement but has its own downside: increased blood loss, difficulty with repair,

Currently, routine episiotomy is *not* recommended, and clinical judgment remains the best guide as to its use. Usually it's to avoid severe tears and to expedite difficult deliveries.

and discomfort postpartum and during sex. And there's no getting around it. A spontaneous tear is likely during most vaginal deliveries, particularly if it's your first. Any good news? Yes! Sutures from any repair are absorbable and won't need to be removed by your doc.

## It Still Hurts!

Where? Most likely it's your perineum, the area between your vagina and rectum that stretches during delivery. You may have had an episiotomy or perineal tear. Any of these causes may make this area feel sore and look swollen and bruised. To ease discomfort and speed healing:

- Apply cold packs or chilled witch hazel pads to the area.
- Take sitz baths; soaking in a few inches of warm water will bring relief.
- Use a water bottle you can squeeze to soothe the area with a stream of warm water after you urinate.
- Use pain medication.
- Always wipe from front to back after you use the toilet to help prevent a healing episiotomy or tear from getting infected with germs from your rectum.

## Why Am I Bleeding?

Even though *lochia* sounds like the name of an exotic orchid, it's not so pretty. Lochia refers to the normal shedding of blood and tissue after delivery. For a few days this vaginal discharge is red brown; then it becomes increasingly watery and pinkish brown for a few weeks. Ultimately, the discharge turns yellowish white. Some women continue to pass lochia for six to eight weeks postpartum. Use sanitary pads rather than tampons at this time.

## ... and Peeing So Much?

Frequent urination is a common complaint during pregnancy, since your kidneys work harder to flush waste products out of your body. In addition, your growing uterus puts pressure on the bladder. Your bladder may be nearly empty, but yes, it still feels like it's full. The weight of your uterus on your bladder may even cause you to leak a little urine when you sneeze or cough. It helps to avoid caffeinated drinks, since they make you urinate more. But don't be tempted to cut out other liquids, since drinking less could lead to dehydration.

I'm worried about giving birth. I've been pretty cool about my pregnancy up until lately, but suddenly I'm realizing that there's a baby that's got to come out and someone is going to have to be there to push it out.

—*a very pregnant Halle Berry*

## I Gave Birth to a Nine-Pound Baby Five Weeks Ago. My V Is Still Very, Very, Very Stretched Out. Will It Ever Return to Its Former Tight Self?

Well, whether or not your vagina returns to its original size depends on several factors: how big your baby is, how many children you've had, and whether you do Kegels (pelvic floor exercises) regularly. After giving birth vaginally, it's normal for the vagina to be larger than it was before, and this effect generally is more pronounced after the birth of a large baby. (Nine pounds definitely qualifies as a large baby!) This is caused by relaxation of the pelvic floor musculature. These muscles will lose their tone with each successive birth, although again, those Kegels can help you tighten them up.

And when you feel discouraged remember: A baby is an angel whose wings decrease while his legs increase.

# C

## Coming Clean: The Dirty Secret About Our Obsession with V Hygiene

*My vagina doesn't need to be cleaned up. It smells good already. Don't try to decorate. Don't believe him when he tells you it smells like rose petals when it's supposed to smell like pussy. That's what they're doing—trying to clean it up, make it smell like bathroom spray or a garden. All those douche sprays—floral, berry, rain. I don't want my pussy to smell like rain. All cleaned up like washing a fish after you cook it. I want to taste the fish. That's why I ordered it.*

—*Eve Ensler*, The Vagina Monologues

Gawd. After watching countless TV commercials and looking at endless glossy magazine ads, you'd think your vagina is a filthy place in dire need of a top to bottom cleaning. *Ha*! That's a big fat V lie. The truth is our bodies naturally possess a delicate balance of yeast and bacteria aimed at keeping our vaginas in tip-top condition. It's awesome. But is that good enough for advertising dudes who want to spread the silly word that we *need* to *buy* products to make our coochies smell sweet? Nah. It's bogus, because too much "cleaning" and seemingly helpful "hygiene" products can actually *cause* itching, irritation, even an infection by disrupting our natural balance of bacteria. Sisters, please listen:

Your vagina does its own cleaning!

That said, the smell of your vagina is directly related to your lifestyle, weight, and diet. Remember, some vaginal discharge is normal; foul odor, copious discharge, itching, or irritation should be a message to get prompt medical attention.

Q. How much money does the average woman spend on feminine hygiene products a year?

A. The average North American woman will spend approximately $120 each year on disposable feminine hygiene products and will use approximately twenty-two feminine hygiene products per period.

## Save Your Money and Your Cha-Cha

**SOAPS**   Nix fragrant soaps or bubble baths because they may cause irritation or allergic reaction. Instead, consider mild soaps like Dove or Ivory. Some find it helpful to use soap only on the vulva and plain warm water on the more delicate vaginal mucus membranes. Vigorous scrubbing with a washcloth or abrasive sponge should be avoided, especially inside the vagina. Pure oils, such as lavender, should be diluted with just a few drops in the tub, since they can also be highly irritating.

**FRAGRANCES/PERFUMES AND FOUL ODORS**  Ladies, it's a fact: The vagina typically has a sweet smell. Under normal circumstances, or even if you have an infection, it's likely that no one else notices an odor from your vagina (except maybe your sexual partner.) As for your period, if you change pads or tampons frequently enough and bathe regularly, no one can smell that either. Feminine sprays, deodorants, and scented tampons are heavily perfumed and can lead to allergic reactions, irritation, and infection. Avoid these. If you have sensitive skin, use a fragrance-free laundry detergent and fabric softener on your undergarments and opt for dye-free TP.

**POWDER, TALC, AND BABY WIPES**  Hey baby, guess what? You're a grown woman. Don't use powders that contain talc: It may be associated with an increased risk of ovarian cancer. Cornstarch and talc-free baby powders are safe, but baby wipes can be *very* irritating for sensitive V's.

**DOUCHING**  The vagina cleanses itself, and that's why douching should probably be avoided altogether. This silly product-driven practice can disturb the natural balance of vaginal organisms; altering your vaginal pH can actually cause pelvic infection. Douching after your period, in fact, can push blood and bacteria into the pelvis. So, DON'T DOUCHE!

The president inserted a cigar into Ms. Lewinsky's vagina, then put the cigar in his mouth and said, "It tastes good."
 —Kenneth Starr

## Simple Tips to Keep Things Balanced

- Do keep your vulva clean and dry; consider using a hair dryer on low or cool when coming out of the shower or tub if you're prone to infection or irritation.
- Don't wear tight-fitting pants or underwear; opt for cotton.
- Don't wear panty hose unless they have a cotton crotch; cut out the crotch altogether if need be.
- Don't use pads or tampons that have deodorant or a plastic coating.
- Do use tampons only if you have your period; choose a tampon that's only as absorbent as you need.
- Don't use perfumed soap or scented toilet paper.
- Don't douche or use feminine sprays or talcs.
- Don't sleep in tight-fitting garments.

# I Don't Use Any Products but My Who-Ha Is Still Off-Balance.

That's because there are other everyday irritants.

**PANTY HOSE/UNDERWEAR**  Yeast and bacteria love moist, dark, nonaerated places. Wearing cotton underwear (or at the very least, cotton crotched) and avoiding thongs and panty hose will allow for more air flow to your V and prevent infection and irritation. Better yet, go commando, especially at night.

**PANTY LINERS/PADS**  Try to avoid these when you don't have your period, since they allow for less airflow to the vagina and may promote infection or skin irritation. Fragrant pads are particularly problematic, since they often cause skin reaction. (As an aside, some women come in with irritation and a rash; on exam, the outline of a pad can be clearly seen on the vulva, like a drawing, making this the obvious source of the problem.)

**SWIMSUITS/WORKOUT CLOTHES**  Try to get out of your wet bathing suit or workout clothes as soon as possible to avoid infection and irritation. Riding a bike or taking spinning classes increases the risk of chaffing; wear a good padded short and consider a gel seat or moisture barrier salve for better cushioning, especially for a lengthy class or long bicycle ride.

# D

## Diaphragm, Ring, Pill, Patch, Sponge, Condom, Cap, IUD, Abstinence, and All the Blah, Blah, Blah About Birth Control

My best birth control these days is just to leave the lights on.

—*Joan Rivers*

Speak to ladies about birth control, and you're likely to hear a heap of horror stories—everything from broken condoms and a surprise trip to Babyville to cranky cups and free flying diaphragms. So, let's get real here. Most of us who need, want, and just *gotta* have birth control (at least for now) want the safest, easiest, most

Just Do Something: One-third of pregnancies in the United States are unplanned!

foolproof method in the whole wide universe. Is that too much to ask? Well, maybe. We all have different needs.

That's why there's not one simple solution for *every* fertile femme on the planet. Since we can't just wish upon a star, maybe the best we can hope for is to learn about each method and make a choice based on the facts that fit our lives.

So, let's look at our options.

## Barrier! Oh, Barrier!

The barrier method prevents pregnancy by providing a barrier between sperm and egg. Duh. But here's something

Yo! Yo! Yo!
Don't Be Silly Protect Your Willy
*Ba-Da-Bing*
Don't Be a Loner Cover Your Boner
*Ba-Da-Bing*

you may not know: Some also protect against STDs. The barrier method includes spermicide, diaphragm, sponge, condom, female condom, and the cervical cap. What's the good news for those who don't like taking hormones? The barrier method doesn't use any. That's why if you're breast-feeding, barrier methods are a good choice.

FYI: Before deciding on any method of birth control, speak with your doctor. Go over the risks of pregnancy involved (they all have some—from 1 percent to much higher), side effects (if any), and instructions.

**SPERMICIDE** This is a chemical that kills sperm. It comes in different forms: foams, films, creams, jellies, and suppositories. You insert spermicide deep into your vagina just before having sexual intercourse. Spermicides provide some pregnancy protection when used alone, but they work much better when combined with the condom, diaphragm, or cervical cap. FYI: Read directions carefully and don't douche!

**DIAPHRAGM**   Seen any UFOs between your legs? Diaphragms are round and dome-shaped reusable latex inserts with a firm but flexible rim that's placed inside your vagina to cover your cervix before sexual intercourse.

## How to Insert Your Diaphragm

1. Wash your hands with soap and water.
2. Inspect the diaphragm for holes.
3. Put approximately 1 tablespoon spermicidal cream or jelly in the cup and around the rim.
4. Sit, squat, lie down, or stand with one foot up on a chair and get comfortable.
5. Separate the lips of the vagina with one hand; pinch the rim of the diaphragm and fold in half with the other hand and insert into the vagina; push it up as far as it will go; the firm part of the rim should be felt behind your pubic bone.
6. Check to see if your cervix is covered by reaching inside; the cervix feels firm like the tip of your nose.
7. A diaphragm can be placed up to six hours prior to sex and must be left in for at least six but no more than twenty-four hours afterward. Do not remove the diaphragm if you have sex more than once within six hours; just insert more spermicidal jelly.
8. Spermicidal jelly should be used with each sex act, no matter how close in time, and no more than two hours prior to sex.
9. For removal, wash your hands with soap and water, hook a finger over the rim, and break the suction, pulling the diaphragm down and out.
10. Upon removing the diaphragm, wash it with warm soap and water and store it in its case.
11. Avoid oil-based lubricants or talc.
12. Avoid use if you have a latex allergy or sensitivity to spermicide.

It must be used with spermicidal cream or jelly. The diaphragm works by blocking the cervix (the opening to the uterus) so that sperm can't enter. Remember: Use your diaphragm at every *conceivable* chance.

**CERVICAL CAP**   This is a small latex cup that you insert into your vagina before sexual intercourse. The cervical cap, which needs to be fitted by a health professional, slips snugly over your cervix. It's smaller than the diaphragm and is used with spermicidal cream or jelly. The cervical cap works by blocking sperm from entering the uterus.

**CONDOMS**   Condoms are thin barriers made of latex, plastic, or natural membranes. They look like long, thin, deflated balloons. There are both male and female condoms. The male condom fits over a man's penis. The female condom fits inside a woman's vagina. Both male and female condoms work by preventing sperm from entering the vagina and reaching an egg.

> One patient described wearing a female condom during sex as sounding like a pack of M&M's ripping open in a movie theater.
> —Dr. D

**SPONGE**   The sponge is a disc-shaped birth control device made of soft foam and is coated with spermicide. It's inserted vaginally to cover your cervix and can be worn for up to thirty hours and put in place up to twenty-four hours before sex. One sponge allows for lots of acts of intercourse in a twenty-four-hour period (yay!). But there's a 16 to 30 percent failure rate (boo!). Don't use the sponge during your period, *if* you're less than six weeks postpartum, *or* you've had toxic shock syndrome in the past.

> Some men are sponge-worthy, and some men are just not sponge-worthy.
> —*Elaine*, Seinfeld

# Hormones! Help! Hormones! Help!

Hormonal methods of birth control include the pill, the ring, the patch, the shot, and the implant. A prescription is required for all of these methods, and none of them protects against STDs.

**ORAL CONTRACEPTION (The Pill)**  When it comes to the pill, there are many brands and formulas available with different levels of estrogen and progestin. Some pills allow for a monthly cycle, while others will give a period every three months or not at all. It prevents pregnancy by stopping ovulation, thickening cervical mucus, and thinning the uterine lining. Talk to your doctor about which pill might be the best one for you. Discuss its side effects. While you're at it, bring up the possibility of taking the mini-pill.

FYI: Fertility returns as soon as you stop taking the pill—like the next day.

**VAGINAL RING (NuvaRing)**  This a flexible plastic ring, easily inserted vaginally, that releases both estrogen and progestin. It's placed for twenty-one days and is removed for seven days, at which time you'll get your period. If you prefer, it can be used continuously and changed every three weeks so that you don't menstruate at all. Follow the instructions carefully.

**PATCH (Ortho Evra)**  The contraceptive patch is a thin plastic—about the size of a matchbook—that you wear on your skin to prevent pregnancy. The patch contains hormones just like the ones in most birth control pills. It releases these hormones through the skin and into the bloodstream. Instead of taking a pill every day, a woman sticks on a new patch each week. The patch works mainly by preventing the ovary from releasing an egg. The failure rate is higher for women over 198 pounds.

FYI: A blood clot may be more likely to develop in women on the patch than on the pill.

**IMPLANT (Implanon)**   This is a progestin-only itty-bitty "rod" inserted under the skin in the upper arm by your health care provider. It works for up to three years and is easily reversible with removal. A big advantage is that you don't have to remember it every day, or even every month. Bonus: You can be sexually spontaneous. Quickie anyone?

**SHOT (Depo-Provera)**   The Depo shot is an every-three-month injection of progestin (DPMA). It also prevents ovulation, thickens cervix mucus, and thins the uterine lining to prevent pregnancy.

Bummer Alert: A lot of women gain weight with the shot.

**IUD**   The IUD is a small, T-shaped piece of flexible plastic that fits inside your uterus to prevent pregnancy. There are two types of IUDs: copper and progestin (a hormone found in birth control pills). The copper IUD lasts ten years and works by interfering with the sperm's ability to reach the egg. The progestin IUD lasts five years and works by thickening cervical mucus and thinning the uterine lining.

**MORNING AFTER PILL (OOPS!)**   *Alert!* This is *not* a contraceptive for regular use. Instead, it's a treatment to prevent pregnancy after unprotected sex. It can be bought over the counter (OTC) if you're eighteen years or older.

Take it *as soon as possible*. Studies show the morning-after pill is most effective if taken within five days of having unprotected sex. This is not an abortion pill.

# You're *Sure* You Don't Want a Baby?

If you're looking for a more permanent solution, there are a few surgical options.

**TUBAL LIGATION**   Having your "tubes tied" is a surgical procedure that cuts, seals, or blocks the fallopian tubes to prevent pregnancy. There is no hormonal change, and the procedure won't change your period or when you'll go through menopause. This is typically an outpatient procedure done in a minimally invasive way; it can also be done at the time of a C-section. Anesthesia is required. Failure rate is less than 1 percent. The risk of ectopic pregnancy (pregnancy found outside the uterus, usually in the fallopian tube) is rare but possible. The procedure is considered permanent, and reversal is not straightforward.

Clueless! Eighteen percent of men believe you can reduce the risk of pregnancy if you have sex standing up.

**TUBAL OCCLUSION**   Tubal occlusion procedures include Essure and Adiana. These allow for a tiny coil to be placed into the fallopian tubes through a telescope (hysteroscope) placed vaginally and then into the cervix and uterus. Scar tissue develops around the coils, causing the tubes to seal shut. This outpatient procedure requires at least a local anesthetic. A confirmatory X-ray type test called an HSG (hysterosalpingram) is done three months later to confirm the tubes are fully blocked. Up to 15 percent of women will need to have the procedure repeated. Like tubal ligation, it won't affect your period or other hormonal changes.

**VASECTOMY**  Vasectomy is a surgical sterilization procedure for guys that cuts or blocks the vas deferens—the tubes that carry sperm from the testes. It's an office procedure done under local anesthesia and takes up to three months to be effective. The failure rate is less than 1 percent.

## Are There Other Options?

**ABSTINENCE**  Well, there's abstinence, choosing to abstain from sexual intercourse, while you still engage in other sexual activities. Some people choose to abstain from all sexual activity. When practiced correctly, abstinence is the only 100 percent surefire method to prevent pregnancy. But it's not much fun.

**PLANNED ABSTINENCE**  This means trying to predict the time of the month when fertility is highest and avoiding sex at that time. Here's how:

**Rhythm or Calendar Method**  This method uses the first day of your last period to determine your most fertile time. In those ladies with a twenty-eight- to thirty-day cycle (from day one of bleeding to day one of bleeding in the next cycle), you should avoid sex from days ten to nineteen. This method is not recommended *if* you have irregular cycles *or* you're nursing.

Want birth control that really works? Every night before we go to bed we spend an hour with our kids.
—*Roseanne Barr*

**Basal Body Temperature**  This method relies on the fact that your morning temperature (taken before you get out of bed), the lowest temperature attained by the body during rest, will rise slightly, 0.5°F, after ovulation. So sex should be avoided from day one of your menses

## What Doesn't Protect You from Pregancy?

**Douching**  Squirting water or any other liquid into the vagina after sex does not kill sperm or prevent pregnancy.

**Plastic wrap instead of a condom**  Plastic wrap or a plastic bag can tear and let sperm escape.

**Urinating right after sex**  Urine does not pass through the vagina, so it does not get rid of the sperm.

**Having sex for the first time**  You can get pregnant even if you've never had sex before.

**A special position**  No matter which way you're standing, sitting, kneeling, etc., if his penis enters—or comes close to—your vagina, *sistah*, you can get knocked up.

until three days after your temperature rises or for about two weeks of the cycle. This won't work *if* you're nursing *or* nearing menopause.

**Monitoring Cervical Mucous**  Cervical mucous is typically more watery and heavier when you're ovulating. To prevent pregnancy, you should avoid sex when watery cervical mucus first appears until three or four days after the heaviest day of mucus.

**WITHDRAWAL**  Also known as coitus interruptus, withdrawal means your man pulls his penis from your vagina before he ejaculates. This won't work *if* he withdraws too late *or* if sperm is released before the big explosion.

**BREAST-FEEDING**  Breast-feeding delays the return of ovulation. That's why it can be somewhat effective in preventing pregnancy, particularly in those who nurse exclusively for the first six months and don't menstruate.

# E

# Egg, Ovulation, and You

It is a well-documented fact that guys will not ask for directions. This is a biological thing. This is why it takes several million sperm cells ... to locate a female egg, despite the fact that the egg is, relative to them, the size of Wisconsin.

—Dave Barry

## Lesson 101: Ovulation! (or Hormonal Cycle/LH Surge)

Well, it's simply the monthly release of an egg from your ovary. In an average twenty-eight-day menstrual cycle, ovulation occurs about fourteen days after the first day of your last period. (Day one is always the first day of your period.) It's like this: Each month an egg matures in a menstruating woman's ovary. The egg is surrounded by a sac called a follicle. The cells of the follicle first produce the hormone estrogen. This triggers a surge of LH (luteinizing hormone) from the pituitary gland in the brain, and the egg is released. The follicle cells then begin to produce progesterone as well as estrogen. This prepares the uterine lining for pregnancy *if* fertilization occurs. If pregnancy does not occur (and depending on where you're at, that's good or bad news), the egg degenerates and the thickened uterine lining sheds and then—you get your period.

Whaaah? A man can smell when a woman is ovulating—and the proof is in his testosterone, says a new study from Florida State University that had undergraduate men sniffing sweaty T-shirts for course credit. The study, published in the journal *Psychological Science*, suggests that olfactory cues signaling a woman's ovulation—her most fertile time—can prime men to have sex with her.

# How Can I Tell When or Even *If* I'm Ovulating?

You can do it. Trust me. Chart your cycle on a calendar for a few months. If you have a regular twenty-eight-day cycle, with day one being the first day of your menses, you'll typically ovulate on or around day fourteen. If you have a shorter or longer cycle, you can count backward fourteen days from when you get your period, and that'll usually be ovulation day. There are a few ways to keep track of your cycle.

### Track Your Symptoms

Most of us will experience one or more of these around the time of ovulation:

- a twinge of discomfort when we ovulate.
- breast soreness.

- just before ovulation, more cervical mucus is produced, and it becomes clear, slippery, and stretchy. Think raw egg white.
- increase in horniness.

### Monitor Your Basal Temperature

It increases about half a degree *after* ovulation. To do this, take your temperature first thing in the morning at the same time every day before you even get out of bed. Chart your temperature on a graph that also shows your menstrual cycle. You should see a pattern of slight temperature increase approximately twenty-four to forty-eight hours after you ovulate. In subsequent months, you can then predict when you'll ovulate.

### Use an Ovulation Predictor Kit or a Fertility Monitor

You can get these kits OTC at most drugstores. They're urine tests that measure your LH. The LH surge predicts ovulation within approximately twenty-four hours. If you want to get pregnant, you should try to have sex every other day for about a week around the time of ovulation—horny or not. To prevent pregnancy, use contraception or avoid sex when you're ovulating.

Really? Ovulating women have more accurate gaydar than the rest of us, according to a study in the *Journal of Psychological Science.* Hmmm...

# I Always Know When I'm Ovulating Because It, Like, *Kills!*

Welcome to the world of *mittelschmerz*. Yeah, it sounds like a German opera, but it literally means "middle pain," and it's the word for the discomfort felt when you're ovulating. For some of us, it's a mild twinge or cramp in the lower belly or back. But for 20 percent of ladies, ovulation is an *intense* pain. The ache can alternate sides, and like clockwork, it happens every month during the midcycle. It can last minutes or hours and usually feels sharp and crampy. Bloating and discomfort can occasionally last for twenty-four to forty-eight hours. You can treat mittelschmerz with ibuprofen a day before you're expecting the discomfort and with a heating pad. Birth control pills are also a common treatment. Why? Well, because they prevent ovulation. If your mittelschmerz symptoms last longer than two or three days, tell your doctor about it, since there might be another reason why you're in pain.

Trouble getting pregnant? You're not alone. The number of American women ages fifteen to forty-four who have ever used infertility services is 7.3 million.

## We've Been Trying for Well Over a Year to Get Pregnant. What's Happening?

Well, that depends. Here's the math: We're born with about 1 to 2 million eggs. By puberty about 300,000 to 400,000 are still there. Of these, about three hundred to four hundred will be ovulated during a woman's reproductive lifetime. You never produce new eggs—*ever*. (Men, on the other hand, produce sperm continuously throughout most of their lives.) Eggs degenerate during pregnancy, with the use of birth control pills, and just naturally as we age, until menopause when they're all gone.

*Ovarian reserve* refers to the number and quality of your eggs and thus to your ability to get pregnant. Since lots of ladies have chosen to delay childbearing for various reasons, ovarian reserve and the testing for it is more relevant than ever before. Sadly, the truth is that *the decline in ovarian reserve is irreversible*. It's affected by:

- Age—over thirty-five years.
- Environmental factors—smoking, history of chemotherapy, or radiation.
- Genetics—family history of early menopause and history of having had ovarian surgery such as ovarian cyst removal or ovary removal.

Testing typically involves blood tests for FSH (a hormone that reflects ovarian function and reserve) and estradiol (a hormone secreted by the ovary that is elevated during ovulation) on day two of your menstrual cycle as well as other more advanced procedures.

## Can It Be Possible That I've Never Ovulated Even Though I Sometimes Get My Period?

Yup. Polycystic ovarian syndrome (PCOS) is a condition in which ovulation doesn't occur or occurs infrequently because of an imbalance in hormones. Sisters with PCOS produce an excess amount of male hormones called androgens. These women usually have irregular menstrual bleeding or no menses at all, and often have trouble getting pregnant. Some have unwanted hair growth in typically male places like the upper lip and chin, between their breasts, on the lower part of the abdomen, and on the inner thighs. Many with PCOS produce too much insulin, and what's produced doesn't work well. This results in

If it's so hard to get pregnant, how do you account for the number of crying children on planes?

—*Samantha*, Sex and the City

obesity and difficulty maintaining and losing weight. The risk of diabetes, uterine cancer, high blood pressure, and heart disease is higher. There are treatments. They include diet, exercise, hair removal, oral antidiabetic medications, and birth control pills. Fertility treatment is often needed to assist with pregnancy.

# F

## Fungus—and Other Infections That Make Us Feel Funky

In response to calls for sexual equality, Pillsbury recently added a new Pillsbury Dough GIRL. Unfortunately, she couldn't come to work. Why? She had a yeast infection. Ha. ha. ha.

Oh why, oh why is the word *fun* in the word *fungus*? The irony! I admit, fungus is not the most tasteful teatime conversation, but let's just deal and get it over with.

Here's the scoop: A small amount of clear or cloudy white fluid passing each day from your V is *totally* normal. Think of this discharge as a lovely moisturizer because, darling, that's what it is. It keeps your lady flower's tissue moist and healthy. And don't fret over a small difference in the amount or color because it usually changes throughout your menstrual cycle and can vary from woman to woman.

(But if you're comparing your discharge with a girlfriend, it may be a little weird, or maybe not. I'm just sayin'.) Anyway, your V normally contains lots of organisms including yeast and bacteria. But sometimes conditions go haywire. Let's take a quick peek at what happens.

**VAGINITIS**  Uh … did you forget that tampon? I'm only asking because a vaginal infection is often the body's reaction to an imbalance in the usual V organisms commonly caused by something foreign inside it. You won't believe how many times women come into my office with a neglected tampon—and believe me—you can smell it a mile away, or more likely from the waiting room. Excuse my candor. Well, it could also be a condom. Other vaginitis triggers are spermicidal or soap, or hormonal changes like menopause or pregnancy. Hey, if you've got itching of the vulva, vagina, or labia; redness, burning, soreness, or swelling of the vulva skin; a stinky odor; foamy, green/yellow, or bloody discharge; pain with sex or urination; abdominal or pelvic pain; think vaginitis and then see your gyno ASAP.

> Use It or Lose It: Regular sexual activity maintains a healthy, juicy, lovely lady flower. If you have a lot of sex with a partner or through masturbation, your V will stay elastic and pliable. Go for it!

**YEAST**  Vaginal yeast infections are caused by a friend you don't want to see—the fungus called candida. It's totally common and mostly visits sisters who have their periods. The usual symptom is an itchy vajayjay. You might also have a thick, white, clumpy vaginal discharge resembling cottage cheese, plus other symptoms like pain while urinating, vulvar soreness or irritation, discomfort with sex, and a red swollen vulva and vagina. You raise your risk for getting yeast with antibiotic use, hormonal contraceptives, and devices like the sponge, diaphragm, or IUD; wearing panty liners or panty hose; using sexual lubricants or sitting around in your wet bathing suit or workout clothes. Yeast infections are also more common if you have a weakened immune system from infection such as HIV or certain medications like steroids or chemotherapy, you're pregnant, or you have diabetes (especially if sugar levels aren't controlled). Even though your yeast infection is not an STD, it's more frequent when you're having sex, especially the oral kind.

Treatment of yeast includes either an oral pill or a topical vaginal treatment with cream or suppository. If it's a simple yeast infection, it'll probably go away in a few days. If you get recurrent infections (more than four a year), you might need treatments repeated. Since vaginal yeast infections are rarely passed from one partner to another, treating your sex partner is generally not recommended. But there are exceptions; I'll treat a partner if symptoms keep recurring.

FYI: Lots of ladies self-treat with OTC medication when they *think* it's yeast. Sometimes you're mistaken, and this can make the right diagnosis for your gyno more challenging—because the wrong treatment can cause further irritation. It's a vicious cycle, frustrating for you—and your doc.

**BACTERIAL VAGINOSIS**  Got BV? Well, it's hard to miss. You'll get the hint because there'll be a noticeable increase in discharge (thin and gray), along with a strong fishy odor. You might also be itchy down there and bleed after sex. What's the cause for all this V havoc? Simply, an imbalance in bacteria types in the vagina that can develop thanks to multiple or new sexual partners, douching, or cigarette smoking. Even though BV is not thought to be an STD, it's more common when you're having sex. BV itself is not harmful, but it can increase the risk of HIV infection and transmission and other STDs, preterm delivery in pregnant women, and postsurgical infection. Your gyno can make a diagnosis and prescribe the proper treatment, which will mean taking antibiotics either orally or intravaginally.

FYI: BV can happen again and again. If that's the case, you'll need more frequent or longer rounds of antibiotics. A good way to avoid all this V drama is to use condoms.

**ATROPHIC VAGINITIS** Add this condition to the list titled "Bummers of Getting Older." You get vaginal atrophy when you stop producing estrogen, and your poor, tired lady flower loses her blossom and elasticity and gets thin and droopy, and, well, dries up. Hold on! It's not *always* menopause doing the damage. It could be lactation, a postpartum period, or anti-estrogenic drugs. And the change in your V doesn't happen overnight. Still, you'll notice it. There might be inflammation, thinning of the vaginal and lower urinary tract tissue, and shortening and narrowing of the V canal, with loss of stretching ease and

### Preadolescent Vaginitis

Preadolescent vaginitis may be the result of infection, congenital abnormality, trauma and sexual abuse, dermatologic conditions, foreign body (toilet paper is the most common), and pinworm, to name a few. Because prepubertal hypoestrogenic tissues are thin and delicate, they're more susceptible to local irritants, foreign bodies, and infection.

*Fungus—and Other Infections That Make Us Feel Funky* 69

less juice. Plus you can be more susceptible to trauma. In other words, you might bleed even during a routine Pap smear. As if that's not enough, there's often itching, burning, infection, painful sex, bleeding, urinary discomfort, and frequency. Your gyno can give you the bad news. *Any* good news? Yes! Your symptoms can be managed by regular use of vaginal nonestrogen moisturizing agents such as Replens and supplemental lubricants during sex: K-Y Jelly or Astroglide. And if you're the right candidate, topical or oral estrogen is an effective treatment.

# G

# Get Down with Your Gyno

Q. What's the diff between a genealogist and a gynecologist?

A. A genealogist looks up your family tree. A gynecologist looks up your family bush!

Too bad you probably don't think there's anything funny about going to the gyno. If you're like most women you have like a million, no! make that like a *gazillion*, reasons *not* to see your gynecologist: You're feeling fat and don't want to be weighed, you might be embarrassed because you have an STI or just *think* you have one (FYI: an excellent reason to be on the examining table!), or you're basically shy, maybe a little uptight, and so showing your lady flower to a doctor is the last thing in the world you want to do. You'd rather bring

For many healthy ladies, a Pap test every two years from ages twenty-one to twenty-nine is sufficient, followed by every three years for women ages thirty to sixty-five.

Jeffrey Dahmer home as your date. Okay, that's extreme, but you get my point—you have *your* reasons. Whatever they are, girl, get over them!

## My Daughter Is Only Thirteen and I Don't Want Her to Visit a Gynecologist Until It's Absolutely, Positively Necessary. How Long Can I Wait?

Yeah, remember when darling Petunia was snug in your arms watching *Beauty and the Beast*? In those days *you* were all that. These days, you're a total embarrassment. According to the recommendation of the American College of Obstetricians and Gynecologists, you should make the first appointment when she's between thirteen and fifteen years old. (Take her sooner if you know she's sexually experienced.) The initial visit won't necessarily include a pelvic examination, but the doctor will provide guidance, preventive services, and screening. The ACOG recommends annual screening for gonorrhea for all sexually active adolescents and for chlamydia in all sexually active women twenty-five and younger. Hopefully, the doc and your

### A Note on Confidentiality

Adolescents may undergo a pelvic examination without their parents' knowledge or permission if the exam is performed for the testing or treatment of a sexually transmitted infection. Laws vary by jurisdiction on confidential access to HIV testing, contraception, and abortion services. Parental consent is required for childhood examinations and adolescent pelvic exams unrelated to sexual contact.

daughter will connect, and she'll contact her gynecologist should any problems pop up in the future.

## Hey What's with That Totally Scary Speculum?

Okay, okay, sure, I get it, but it can't be helped. Gynecologists need to use a speculum to look inside your vagina and see your cervix clearly. Squeamish Alert: Ready? There's a wide variety of vaginal specula (metal or plastic) that can be used by a gynecologist to perform an examination. Most of these devices have two blades (not at all sharp!) and a handle. Once the blades are clicked into place, the handle can be locked by fastening a screw. It helps to breathe deeply if you're feeling anxious. Who wouldn't be?

> Then she took out a speculum the size of a milk shake machine.
> —*Tina Fey*, Bossypants

## My Gynecologist Is Always Asking Me a Million Questions before I Even Spread My Legs. Is This Normal or Is She Just Being Nosey?

Sounds as if you have a good gynecologist, so don't hold back. Blab on! The more information your physician has, the better she or he can treat you.

When you go to the gyno, here's what you *should* be asked:

- The reason for your visit; your age; your obstetrical history, which includes info about prior pregnancies (Vaginal or cesarean deliveries? Miscarriages, abortions, any complications or

## Why to Go to the Gyno (Besides Your Annual)

- Vaginal discharge
- Pain
- Breast problems
- Problems getting pregnant
- Abnormal bleeding
- Urinary complaints
- Sex issues

unique circumstances that are pertinent to each?). You should also be questioned about your menstrual history (age at first menses or menopause, cycle regularity, flow amount and length, issues with cramps or abnormal bleeding habits, issues with hot flashes or night sweats, whether you use tampons or pads, any problems inserting those tampons?). Stay put; we're not done yet...

- You should also be asked about prior Pap smears and results or treatments for irregularities. Have you had prior or frequent infections or STDs, ovarian cysts, uterine fibroids, polyps, endometriosis, polycystic ovaries, or DES exposure? Any trouble with urinating or moving your bowels? And we're still not done...

- On to your sexual history: Are you currently having sex? If so, with men, women, or both? Do you have multiple partners? What do you use for contraception (past and present)? Is sex painful? Do you suffer from vaginal dryness? Do you have libido or orgasm issues?

- What medications do you take, including prescription meds, OTC meds, vitamins, or supplements? Do you have allergies to any medications?

- Then there's your general medical history: Do you have any current or past issues with the heart, lungs, thyroid, kidney, liver, bleeding or clotting problems, psychiatric problems, or any prior hospitalizations, and if so for what? Have you had surgery before? Let's take a breather.... Onward.

- Now for your lifestyle habits: Do you smoke and if so how much? Do you drink alcohol and if so how much? Do you use drugs? Are you married, single, partnered, divorced, or widowed? Are you the victim of any abuse? Are you a student or do you work, and if so what do you do? Do you exercise regularly?

> Your OB/GYN should always (NO EXCEPTIONS) be sensitive and nonjudgmental. Nothing is off-limits. In my practice, I've heard or seen it all ... really!
> —Dr. D

- Your doctor will also want to have a picture of your family history, specifically whether there are female cancers in the family (parents, grandparents, siblings) or a pattern of cancers in your family line. And your gynecologist will want to know about immediate family with blood clots or heart disease.

## What Should a Good Annual Exam Be Like?

Typically, a nurse or assistant will take your weight (in my office, women will remove belts, shoes, clothes, and even jewelry to be weighed. Wedding rings? Yes!), blood pressure, pulse, and temperature. Your doc or nurse practitioner may also check your skin for rashes, discoloration, and temperature; your neck for enlarged glands and thyroid gland for enlargement or nodules (hard, roughly spherical abnormal structures). A breast exam is also typically done, first in the sitting position and then lying down to check for symmetry, pain, lumps, skin changes, nipple discharge, and armpit lumps. Your physician should also feel your abdomen for pain, masses, or enlarged organs.

Lesbians may be at higher risk for certain cancers (colon, lung, uterine, ovarian, and breast) and cardiovascular disease and diabetes, but in general should be screened according to standard guidelines. FYI: STDs can be transmitted between women.

The actual pelvic exam may take only about five minutes—not long at all. The entire time you're in the exam room, including the question and answer session with your provider, may take up to forty-five minutes, especially if you have questions or are seeking a contraceptive method.

## I Never Know What My Doctor Is Doing Down There.

You're lying on the exam table with your feet in stirrups feeling totally exposed and vulnerable? Hello, cowgirl! You're getting a pelvic exam. I've done several thousand of them, so let me tell you about it: first, your external V is inspected carefully, including the pubic hair distribution, skin, labia (minora and majora), clitoris, urethral opening, and the various glands, hymen or hymeneal remnants, and anus.

Debatable: A male gynecologist is like an auto mechanic who has never owned a car.
—*Carrie P. Snow*

Now for the "fun" part: a speculum is *gently* (note the adverb!) inserted into your vajayjay to check out your

## Possible Tests

Certain tests may be taken, including a Pap smear with or without an HPV test, cultures for infection, and blood and urine tests. In addition, your gyno may order or perform a mammogram, ultrasound of the breasts or pelvis, and a bone density test, and recommend immunizations or consults with other docs.

vaginal walls and cervix and take swabs for infection and, if needed, a Pap test. Next, a *bimanual exam* is done in which your gyno inserts one or two fingers of one hand vaginally to elevate your pelvic organs while she or he uses the other hand on the abdomen to sweep the organs downward to inspect the cervix, uterus, and ovaries and feel for size, pain, mobility, and consistency. Had enough? Maybe not. A rectal exam is occasionally done to feel the back of uterus and ovaries and to check for rectal irregularities, blood in the stool, and pelvic masses in those too young to tolerate a vaginal exam.

# H

## Hormones, Hot Flashes, and Jalapeño Peppers

If scientists ever find a cure for menopause, our big problem will be global cooling.

*—Anonymous*

Menopause is a touchy subject for lots of us careening toward what could be bumpy terrain. Of course, some lucky sisters are clueless and breeze along. But let's not talk about *them* right now, since there are 19 million American women driving through menopause this year. For plenty of ladies, it will feel like maneuvering a Mack truck. Hold on to that wheel!

I've got Postmenopausal Zest!
*—Margaret Mead*

### So, What *Is* Menopause?

Okay, let me explain without any hype: It's a time in your life, usually between the ages of forty-five and fifty-five, when your ovaries stop producing estrogen and your menstrual period ends. The average age of menopause is fifty-one years. Sound simple? Well, there are also other terms sometimes used to describe the time before and after you stop menstruating. Here you go:

**PERIMENOPAUSE (The Menopause Transition)** This stage starts when your menstrual periods first begin to change. They can become more or less frequent with more or less bleeding, including skipped periods. This transition can last for a few years.

**MENOPAUSE** Doctors clinically diagnose menopause as twelve months of amenorrhea (no period) in a woman over forty if there aren't any other causes.

**POSTMENOPAUSE** This is the time after menopause.

# Is There Any Way to Know *When* I'm Going to Go through Menopause?

Got a crystal ball? Actually you won't need one. There are factors that can affect its timing.

**GENETIC** If the women in your family have gone through an early menopause, you're also at a higher risk for doing it sooner.

**LIFESTYLE** The age of menopause is reduced by about two years in women who smoke.

# I Think I'm In It; What Should I Do Next?

Don't murder your partner. Only kidding ... sorta.

Seriously, if you're over forty and haven't had a menstrual period in twelve months, there's a good chance you're menopausal. Most women don't need lab testing to confirm it, especially if you're having symptoms such as hot flashes or vaginal dryness. Hormonal lab tests such as FSH or estradiol may be helpful in diagnosis, but won't necessarily give a surefire answer because these test values vary month-to-month during perimenopause.

> There are only three female animals known to have menopause: elephants, humpback whales, and human females.

# I've Had a Hysterectomy. Will I Go through Menopause?

After a hysterectomy when you no longer have a uterus (but still have ovaries), it can be tougher to know if you're menopausal because you're not menstruating. You might develop menopausal symptoms as your ovaries stop working and your blood levels of estrogen begin to fall. If you have bothersome symptoms of menopause after a hysterectomy, give your doctor a holler.

> Yo! You're not alone. By 2013, 50 million women in the U.S. will be in menopause.

# My Period Is So Wacky! I Just Want to Know If It's Normal.

A majority of ladies begin to notice changes in their periods during perimenopause. Relax, changes are normal and include:

- Having your period more or less often than usual. A typical cycle length is twenty-one to thirty-five days.
- Bleeding for fewer days than before.
- Skipping one or more periods.

If you're less than forty-five years old and you stop having periods, or if you have questions about menopausal symptoms, speak to your doctor. You may need further testing to see if another issue, including pregnancy, is the reason for your symptoms.

Irregular vaginal bleeding may be a normal part of menopause, or it may be a sign of pregnancy, thyroid disease, or something else. If you're concerned, it's another reason to check in with your gyno.

## How Can I Tell If I'm Bleeding Too Much?

Sometimes it's hard to know whether you're on overflow. It's a good idea to see your doctor if:

- You're bleeding more often than every three weeks.
- It's excessive and interfering with your life.
- It's between periods—even if only spotting.
- It's after menopause (even if it's just a dot).
- It's after sex.

## I'm in Perimenopause: Do I Still Need Birth Control?

Don't dump your diaphragm or birth control pills *yet*. Sure, you're less likely to get pregnant after forty-five years, but it's possible—especially if you're still having occasional periods and sex regularly. And, dudette, if you don't want to be pregnant, you should continue to use some form of birth control until you're positively menopausal. Wishful thinking doesn't count.

## Hot Flashes

Sizzling bolts of fire typically begin as the sudden sensation of heat centered on your upper chest and face and spread fast through your body. This burning sensation can last from two to four minutes, is often associated with profuse perspiration and occasionally palpitations, and is sometimes followed by chills and shivering, and a feeling of anxiety. And don't think they're just a flash in the pan. Hot flashes usually occur several times a day; some women get only one or two each day to as many as one per hour during the day and night. Flashes are common at night and frequently interfere with sleep. But hey, some women don't get any! Keep in mind—the following stoke hot flashes:

Red-hot mama? Not for long. Eighty percent of women who experience hot flashes are over the hump within eighteen to twenty-four months.

- Smoking
- High body mass index: Overweight women are more, not less, likely to have hot flashes.
- Less physical activity
- Stress

Here are some easy and supercool ways to stop hot flashes:

- Dress in layers. Don't wear wool or synthetics and be wary of silk. Avoid turtlenecks and stick to open-neck shirts.
- Keep ice water on hand and nix hot beverages. Substitute soft drinks for alcohol.

- Reduce or eliminate chocolate and coffee.
- Pass on jalapeños! Also avoid cayenne, chile peppers, wasabi, and hot mustard.
- Eat smaller, more frequent meals rather than large ones.
- Lower the thermostat.
- Wear cotton pajamas, a nightgown, or just your birthday suit to bed.
- Use cotton, not synthetic, sheets.
- Get a bigger bed if you and your partner are on different heat planets.
- Take a cool shower before bed.
- Leave the bed and stick your head in the freezer. Trust me!

## It Feels Like I Have a Fever at Night, and My Sheets Get Soaked. What's Going On?

When hot flashes happen during sleep, they're called night sweats. These steamy "darlings" may make you perspire through your clothes and wake up because you're either hot or cold (because the sweat is evaporating). It can happen one or more times a night. And truthfully, Ms. Groggy, waking frequently can make it tough to get a good night's sleep, which is crucial for your mental and physical well-being. Thank your crummy night's sleep if you develop other problems such as fatigue, irritability, trouble concentrating, and mood swings. It can be nightmare.

In the Western world, about 75 to 85 percent of women experience hot flashes; in contrast, only about 12 percent of Japanese women and 30 percent of Nigerian women report having experienced hot flashes.

## OMG, I'm So Dry Down There.

Well, sadly, that's one of the side effects of menopause. As levels of estrogen in your blood fall, tissues inside your vagina and urethra can become thin and dry. But you can get juicy *without* hormones:

- Boost your water intake.
- Avoid fragrances and chemicals in personal products.
- Eat soy and other "plant estrogen" containing foods.
- Try a personal lubricant from over the counter, vitamin E vaginal supplements, or olive oil.

Caveat: Most suggestions require a few weeks to work, so remember to be patient!

## I Once Loved to Have Sex, Now I Couldn't Care Less! What's Wrong With Me?

Probably nothing. Vaginal dryness can lead to pain with sex. And just the fear of this pain can result in a lower sex drive. Good news! Some women report regaining their sex drives once they are postmenopausal even without replacement hormones. Why? No fear of pregnancy and no issues with that time of the month!

## Why Am I on an Emotional Roller Coaster?

Some ladies develop problems with mood, such as sadness, difficulty concentrating, feeling uninterested in normal activities, and sleeping too much or having trouble staying asleep. Try getting plenty of natural sunlight (don't forget the sunscreen!), avoid alcohol, get some exercise, and

### Oh No, What Else Can I Expect During Menopause?

**Balance Issues**   You can probably blame an estrogen deficiency if you're off-kilter during menopause.

**Skin Changes**   Collagen in the skin and bones is reduced by estrogen deficiency and can lead to aging and wrinkling of the skin.

**Joint Pain**   Some women experience diffuse joint pain during menopausal transition and the postmenopausal period.

**Menstrual Migraines**   These headaches cluster around the onset of each menstrual period. Women hope they'll stop once they go through menopause, but no such luck. In many women, these headaches worsen in frequency and intensity during the transition.

**Breast Pain**   Tenderness and pain are common during early menopause, but begin to lessen in the later transition.

try talk therapy with friends or a professional. Let your doctor know if you're experiencing more than the blahs.

## How about Hormone Replacement Therapy?

Okay, so you've probably heard the controversy swirling around hormone replacement therapy (HRT) for menopause-related symptoms. As the number of health risks associated with HRT grows, docs are less likely to prescribe it, and plenty of sisters are discontinuing its use. That said, get the facts first and then discuss your individual situation with your gyno.

Celebrate! October 18 is World Menopause Day.

### So, Are There *Any* Benefits to HRT?

Women who opt for standard hormone therapy during menopause are typically prescribed estrogen and progestin. The most common reason to take hormone therapy is to treat those loathsome menopausal symptoms we've been talking about. Other benefits include protection from osteoporosis, colorectal cancer, and symptoms of vaginal atrophy.

Caution: You should *not* take hormone replacement if you have a history of blood clots, breast cancer, or heart disease. Don't consider taking hormones if menopausal symptoms aren't bothering you. Speak with your doctor about alternatives.

### Is There Any Way to Reduce HRT's Risks?

- Minimize the amount of medication you take. If you do take hormones, use the lowest effective dose for the shortest amount of time needed to treat symptoms.
- Find the best delivery method for you. You can take estrogen in the form of a pill, patch, gel, vaginal cream, or ring.
- Use progestin. If you haven't had a hysterectomy and you're using estrogen therapy, you'll also need progestin to protect you from developing uterine cancer.

### Are There Any Medications Besides HRT That Help?

- SSRI'S, antidepressants such as Prozac, Zoloft, and Lexapro.

- Anti-anxiety meds such as Xanax can reduce anxiety and help with sleep. FYI: These meds are habit forming. Use with caution.
- Clondine, an antihypertensive pill or patch that can relieve hot flashes.
- Progesterone may help reduce hot flashes.

## My Friend Is Using Bioidentical Hormone Therapy. Does It *Really* Work?

Bummer Alert: There's no evidence that these products are any safer or more effective than traditional HRT. Bioidentical hormones have a chemical structure similar to the hormones that the human body naturally produces. The treatment involves individualized doses of natural compounded estrogen and progestins, and come in pills, gels, sublingual tablets, even suppositories. Speak with your doctor about what it involves.

## What About Phytoestrogens?

Big word but not a big help. Plant-derived estrogens are called phytoestrogens. They've been marketed as a "safer" alternative to hormones for women with menopausal symptoms. The effectiveness of supplements containing phytoestrogens, such as red clover, black cohash, or evening primrose oil, is questionable, although some women claim anecdotally that they help. Women who've had breast cancer should avoid phytoestrogens. Phytoestrogens are found in so many healthful foods—better to load up on soybeans, tofu and other dietary soy, and chickpeas, lentils, flaxseed, grains, fruits, and vegetables!

More than 30 percent of women say they use herbs and other supplements to deal with their symptoms, according to the North American Menopause Society.

# I

# *Inside Info on Intercourse Snafus*

There are approximately 100 million acts of sexual intercourse each day.

According to surveys, the Americans and Greeks top the list at 124 and 117 times each year, respectively. The Indians do it only 76 times a year, while the Japanese seem to be the least interested, clocking in at a lowly 6 times annually!

## ... and How Many of Those Intimate Encounters Are Awesome?

Rather than beat around the *bush*, if having sexual intercourse is no longer fun—or was never a bowl of cherries—it could be:

**VAGINAL DRYNESS** It can happen at *any* age, although it's most common in postmenopausal women. Here are some reasons why we go dry:

- Declining estrogen level
- Inhibited desire
- Inadequate foreplay
- Medications such as antihistamines, antidepressants, and antihypertensives
- Medical disorders such as diabetes

Now for the good news—dry can be managed! Here are some tips on how to get wet:

- Increase foreplay to give more time for natural lubrication.
- Hold off penetration until you're driven mad by yearning.
- Try OTC vaginal moisturizers and lubricants, either daily vaginal moisturizers like Replens that don't contain hormones, or an OTC lubricant to use during sex such as K-Y Jelly, Astroglide, or Silk-E. Follow directions.
- Give natural lubricants like vegetable oil, egg whites, or saliva a whirl.
- In a pinch, try oil-based products such as petroleum jelly or mineral oil, which can damage condoms or diaphragms but are otherwise reasonable options.
- Avoid perfumed body or hand lotions, which may be irritating to the vagina.

No Matter How You Say It: To screw, bang, reproduce, copulate, pork, booger, hump your honey, get laid, lay some pipe, hide the salami, to slam (or to get slammed), bury the bone, stuff the donut, moisten the carpet, dine in the Y, to munch on the rug, slam the hen, shoot the sherbet, or whack Willy Wonka into Wonderland...

- Speak with your gyno about vaginal estrogen, which requires a prescription and may not be right for every woman. Vaginal estrogen comes in various forms.
- Consider an estrogen cream. The upside is it works for both vaginal and vulvar discomfort. But it can be way messy, and since it's absorbed into your bloodstream, it has potential side effects such as increased risk of breast cancer, uterine cancer, and blood clots.
- Speak with your gyno about Vagifem, a small vaginal estrogen tablet inserted twice weekly, or Estring, a flexible vaginal ring worn inside the vagina for three months at a time. Both claim minimal to no absorption into the bloodstream—and therefore—less risk.

**SEMEN ALLERGY**   Sometimes sisters complain about itching, burning, swelling, and redness and, much less commonly, shortness of breath, rash, and hives, around an hour after sexual intercourse. On exam there's no sign of infection, skin condition, or reaction to a particular product. In these unusual cases, patients have asked, "Could I be allergic to my partner?" The short answer is yes—and most often women under forty years old with a family history of major allergic reactions are complaining. Talk about an intimacy obstacle. Since symptoms won't occur if condoms are used, that's one way to prevent it. Another, in severe cases, is medication. Speak with your doc.

Remember: Use it or lose it! Sexual activity, including masturbation, may help the vaginal tissues remain elastic and soft and prevent narrowing and discomfort.

**VAGINISMUS**   Vaginismus is the tightening and spasm of the muscles at your V's opening. This involuntary muscle contraction can make it painful, difficult, or virtually impossible to have vaginal intercourse. In fact, vaginismus can also make putting in a tampon or a pelvic exam tough going. You can get your lady flower to blossom with physical therapy and relaxation exercises. Vaginal dilators that gradually increase in size may also help.

Diet Delight: Sex can burn about 70 to 120 calories for a 130-pound woman and 77 to 155 calories for a 170-pound man every hour.

**VULVODYNIA**   This is an unprovoked stinging, burning, irritation, rawness, or pain anywhere on the vulva with no other obvious cause. Your gyno will diagnose your condition based on your history, a physical exam, and by canceling out all the other usual suspects. Treatment is an individual matter. It may include application of topical anesthetic jelly ten minutes before sexual intercourse (don't forget to wipe away the excess prior to sex so your partner's penis won't get numb!), meticulous hygiene, hypoallergenic lubricants, physical therapy, Botox injections, antidepressants, analgesics (pain meds), nerve blocks, and of course emotional support and counseling. Vulvar ice packs are also soothing after sex. You can find more helpful information through the National Vulvodynia Association at www.nva.org.

YA THINK? No woman needs intercourse; few women escape it.
—Andrea Dworkin

**DEEP PAIN**   Deep pain during intercourse could signal other issues, so discussing it with your gyno is essential. Sometimes, pain felt deep inside during sex might be due to your individual anatomy and can be managed by

## Hysterectomy and Sexual Intercourse

Hysterectomy, which is the surgical removal of the uterus, does not *generally* doesn't affect sexual function after you've healed. But here's a caveat: Removal of your ovaries will deplete estrogen, and then dryness occurs. Some surgeons and patients feel that not removing the cervix during hysterectomy may make for better sexual function and pelvic support. Here's the conundrum: The reason for hysterectomy may affect one's sex life more than the surgery itself. It's personal. Women undergoing surgery for cancer may be depressed, fatigued, and facing further treatment. Others are so happy and relieved to have treated heavy bleeding or large fibroids, for example, that with hysterectomy they feel liberated and actually have better sex lives after the operation.

simply changing positions. For example, if your uterus is tilted, military position may be uncomfortable but being on top could feel loads better. Or it could be one of these conditions:

**Pelvic Inflammatory Disease (PID)**   PID is an infection of the uterus, fallopian tubes, and nearby pelvic structures, which can cause scar tissue and chronic pelvic pain including pain during sex. Treatment involves antibiotics and at times surgery.

**Ovarian Cysts**   Diagnosis is made by history, physical exam, and ultrasound. Treatment may include medication, birth control pills (which can suppress ovarian cysts), or surgery for definitive removal.

**Fibroids**   These are benign muscular growths on the uterus or cervix; they're common and a frequent cause of discomfort during sex. For some, fibroids are small and no problem. Other women hold off on treatment because fibroids usually shrink in menopause. But in some cases fibroids cause unmanageable symptoms, including heavy bleeding or pain or interference with sex. In these cases, options include surgical removal with myomectomy (removal of fibroids only) or hysterectomy (removal of the uterus with fibroids), or embolization, an invasive procedure to diminish the blood supply to the uterus in an effort to shrink fibroids.

**Endometriosis**   This is a condition in which cells that typically line the uterus are found on your ovaries, fallopian tubes, and other pelvic structures. This tissue then bleeds monthly because of hormonal changes and can cause scarring, pain, and problems getting pregnant. Diagnosis is made by history, physical exam, and at times laparoscopy.

**Genital Prolapse**   Genital prolapse is when the cervix, uterus, vagina, bladder, or rectum are bulging inside or protruding from the vagina. The condition usually occurs when the pelvic floor muscles relax, in part as a result of childbirth. While Kegel exercises may help in mild cases, surgical intervention may be necessary with more severe cases. A common treatment option for prolapse includes insertion of a pessary, which is a firm rubber device with support, to hold the organs inside. Unfortunately, such a device means sexual intercourse is O-U-T.

Sisters with V abnormalities from birth or because of trauma, or women who have undergone female circumcision, may benefit from surgical treatment to enhance the vagina for better sexual function. Sexual abuse is associated with chronic pelvic pain and sexual pain disorders. If this is true for you, seek counseling and therapy. There's an excellent chance you can be helped.

# J

## Jive and Jumping to the Wrong Conclusions

Definition of JIVE: to irritate or annoy; to throw off someone's style; pointless or deceptive talk/rhetoric

"Quit jivin' me, turkey."
"Don't give me that jive."

—*Urban Dictionary*

Ya-da, ya-da, ya-da. Sisters love to talk. We share our deepest secrets, and we're quick to offer advice and all the know-how about what we know about—and what we really don't know about. That's a big part of what brings us together, keeps us solid, and makes us cool. But stuff goes wrong: Sometimes a personal anecdote becomes dyed-in-the-wool truth when, in fact, it's only *one* woman's personal story. Or it's really only "truthiness," as the late-night satirist Stephen Colbert might say. Meaning, there's a trace of fact, but it's pretty muddy. Or we repeat the same old wives' tales we heard from our mothers. Not that we're dissing our mothers. *Puh—leeeze*. It's more like the old game of telephone: Info gets distorted the more it's repeated. So let's take care of all this misinformation here and now.

These are some of the most common misconceptions that come up over and over again in Dr. D's day-to-day practice.

# Birth Control Pill Jive

### You Need to Take a Break from the Birth Control Pill at Least Once a Year

Heck no. Many women can safely stay on the pill until menopause without a break.

### Using the Pill May Make It Harder to Get Pregnant in the Future

Relax. The pill won't harm your fertility or prevent you from getting pregnant in the future. A couple of caveats: If you went on the pill to control irregular cycles, you might still have irregular cycles when you get off the pill. For this reason, you might have trouble conceiving because you may have a preexisting ovulation issue. If you're over thirty-five or forty when you stop taking the pill, your fertility is likely to have declined because of age. Eggs last only so long!

Q: Are birth control pills deductible?
A: Only if they don't work.

### You Need to Wait at Least Three Months After Coming Off the Pill to Conceive

Nah. You don't have to wait any specific amount of time after stopping the pill to conceive safely. The only reason it may be recommended to wait three months is that it could take that long for your cycle to regulate, and it may be easier to date your pregnancy. But the truth is there's no harm in trying right away.

### It's Unsafe to Use the Pill to Manipulate Your Cycle
It's perfectly safe, and docs have been recommending this method for years, for example, if you don't want to get your period on your wedding day, honeymoon, vacation, or athletic event.

FYI: You can occasionally get breakthrough bleeding when manipulating your pills.

### The Pill *Always* Causes Huge Weight Gain
Here's an example of truthiness: *Most ladies won't gain weight on the pill.* If you do, it's probably because you're retaining water, and it's usually no more than two to three pounds. Many girls start the pill during adolescence, which is a time when healthy young women gain some weight anyway. So, in this instance, packing on the pounds is just a timely coincidence. Finally, some women find the pill bumps up their appetite, and if they don't pump up the willpower, they could be digging into a nightly bag of chips. If this is your scenario, ask your gyno to try switching you to a different brand of birth control pill.

## Miscellaneous Jive

### You Can't Get Pregnant If a Man Pulls Out Prior to Ejaculation
Don't take any chances. It's possible there's sperm in the pre-ejaculate fluid your guy secretes before he climaxes.

## Using Lubricant Will Help You to Get Pregnant

This is totally false. Some lubricants can actually *prevent* you from getting pregnant. If you're really dry and trying to conceive, be creative. Opt for egg white or vegetable oil, rather than a commercial lubricant.

> The priceless galaxy of misinformation called the mind.
> —*Djuna Barnes*

## You Shouldn't Exercise or Do Strenuous Activity During Your Period

Just do it. There's no harm in exercising while you've got your period. Bonus points: It may even help with cramps.

## Condoms Prevent the Transmission of *All* STDs

While you're less likely to get an STD when condoms are used, you're still vulnerable to transmission. HPV and herpes in particular can be spread by direct contact with areas not covered by the condom.

Still, don't be a fool, vulcanize the tool.

## Only Women Who've Had Casual Sex Can Get STDs

Seriously, you only have to have unprotected sex ONE time just ONCE with ONE partner who's had other partners to potentially be exposed to STDs. And remember: Some STDs can be spread via oral and anal sex as well as skin-to-skin contact.

## In a Monogamous Relationship, an HPV Diagnosis Always Means Someone Has Cheated

Stop the divorce papers! An HPV diagnosis may be the result of persistent HPV infection from years (even decades ago) rather than a new exposure.

## If You Have An IUD You Can't Use Tampons

An IUD does not interfere with tampons.

## Intercourse During Pregnancy Is Dangerous for the Baby

Intercourse is safe during pregnancy—unless your doc has nixed it. Your babe is well protected inside your muscular uterus and is cushioned in cozy fluid.

## The Morning-After Pill Causes Abortions

In fact, emergency contraception prevents pregnancy by blocking fertilization and implantation. It does not induce abortions.

## If You're a Virgin, Your Hymen Will Break

Sure, some women "break" their hymen when they first have intercourse—but lots of other sisters break theirs by bike riding or horseback riding or some other less common way. And you don't always bleed profusely, either.

## Simultaneous Orgasm Is a Must for a Great Sex Life

No way. Women can see stars, hear whistles blowing, and fly to the metaphorical moon while having orgasm after orgasm, or enjoy sex to the max without even having an orgasm. One thing is for sure: It really doesn't depend on synchronicity.

# K

# Killer Exercises and V Infection

How can exercise be bad for you? Well, we'll tell you how ...

V-straddle injuries can happen because of bike riding, horseback riding, zip-lining, or spinning. Fall flat on your V, and hematomas (collections of blood), bruises, and significant lacerations can happen. These boo-boos are usually just treated with TLC, which includes ice packs for twenty-four hours, compression, rest, and sitz baths. If you've *really* done a number on your who-ha, an examination under anesthesia, stitches, or more extensive surgical repair may be needed. Sure, less serious vulvar and vaginal cuts and bruises can be frightening because they bleed a lot. And vulvar hematomas are scary because some can expand to grapefruit size or even bigger. But no worries: Believe it or not, most will resolve spontaneously. In a rare case, your doctor may have to drain it with surgery.

Strange but True: Changing a light bulb can cause damage to your lady flower! While a patient was standing on a chair to change a light bulb, she fell, hitting her V on the back post of the chair!

General rule: Hydrate well and get out of damp and wet workout clothes and swimsuits as soon as possible to avoid vulvar infection, irritation, and V infection.

## I've Been Training for a Century Bike Ride, and It's Really Bothering My V Area. I Swear I'm Not Only Feeling Sore, I'm *Getting* Sores!

Oooh, irritation, discomfort, and at times pressure sores (with cracked and broken skin or blisters) can happen to your poor vulva thanks to cycling. Not surprisingly, some of us call it being "saddle sore." Girl, it can be a pain in the ass. I mean—pain in the vajayjay. Prevention is in order: Padded chamois shorts are a *must* whenever you're cycling or spinning. Consider a gel seat cover for more padding and cushioning. An open seat with V cutout or groove may help prevent pressure sores. A biking balm, such as Chamois BUTT'r or Bodyglide can be applied to high-friction areas or shorts to limit chafing and reduce saddle sores—especially if you're going on a long ride. Happy trails!

## What about Running?

Are we talking chafing here? This is a real problem for runners, especially in warm weather or with longer distances. Sweaty clothing or skin rubbing against skin can cause painful stinging or burning and a red rash. It's most common around the groin and inner thighs—and the *nipples*. (Okay, so nipples aren't related to the V, but chafing there is really awful and common, so it's worth mentioning.) Tighter-fitting and moisture-wicking or cotton clothing will help prevent chafing. Before running, try A&D ointment, Vaseline, cornstarch, or udder balm (off-label, typically used for cow udders; we're not saying you're a cow but hey, it works). Smearing the product on your vulva may be an effective preventative.

## I Think Swimming Is Giving Me a Yeast Infection

I'll bet you're staying in your wet bathing suit for an extended period of time, perhaps lolling poolside with a piña colada in hand? Well, while you're enjoying yourself, a vulvar and vaginal infection or irritation can be developing. Get out of that suit and into something dry and sexy before you schmooze! Oh, and while we're on the subject of swimming, don't worry about swimming while you're menstruating. That shouldn't cause a problem. And forget those old wives' tales: It's unlikely that menstrual blood will attract sharks while scuba diving or snorkeling.

# L

## Labioplasty, Vaginoplasty, and Ever Lovin' V Vanity

Lawrence of my labia!
— *Samantha Jones*, Sex and the City

It's the new world of designer vaginas: the latest entry into cosmetic surgery. We've already nipped, tucked, implanted, and vacuumed every other part of our bodies, and now some sisters are turning their quest for perfection to their genitals. Elective surgeries that promise a better sex life or more aesthetically pleasing private parts are on a gallop. But both the medical community and cultural busybodies are divided over whether these are valid, beneficial surgeries or just over-the-top who-ha obsessions. *You* decide.

Labia shapes and sizes are remarkably variable, and there really is no "normal." But if you want to get technical, the typical labia is less than 2 inches wide.

# Help! I *Hate* My Labia. It Looks Fat! Can I Put It on a Diet?

Sorry. Eliminating fried foods and Gummi bears from your daily diet won't do it. But you're not alone in thinking your labia is chubby. More women than ever before are coming into my office worried their labia is too fat, uneven, wrinkly, saggy, or unsightly. Whether it's a misguided judgment call or the real deal is relative. First things first: Compassion and empathy are in order.

Listen to common complaints:

I hate wearing a bathing suit or anything spandex like yoga pants because it looks like there's a pillow between my legs.

I have to fold up my labia and push it into my vagina so the bulge isn't huge.

Nothing slips into my vagina easily—especially tampons or penises. Why? Because of these floppy lips!

It's not wholly about L-looks. Sisters can suffer from chronic irritation, infection, poor hygiene, and pain during sex or sports because of their flabby labia. And there's the emotional and psychological stress, too. Some women just don't feel "beautiful or feminine enough down there." This is particularly heartbreaking in vulnerable teens, who, for example, might be too embarrassed to change in the locker room. Sometimes counseling and education about personal hygiene and clothing choices helps overcome the anxiety and dissatisfaction. But an increasing number of women are opting for surgery.

**LABIOPLASTY** The vast majority of complaints involve the labia minora, and this cosmetic procedure reduces the dimensions of labia minora (camel toe) or the labia majora. Complications are rare but can include infection, bleeding, scarring, pigment changes, painful sex, or other poor cosmetic results. Less commonly, if the labia majora (outer lips) are "bulky and bulging," surgical removal of fatty tissue or liposuction is an option. In other cases, when women complain of a "sagging and wrinkly" labia majora (because of advancing age or childbirth or massive weight loss), collagen injections or autologous fat transplant (donation of fat from another area on your own body) may be the way to go. Laser treatments are another avenue to explore.

"The New View" campaign based in New York City is a feminist organization of social scientists and clinicians that oppose labioplasty. They claim these procedures are turning healthy female sexuality into a medical problem, thereby endangering women's health just for profit.

## Botox Worked Wonders on My Forehead Wrinkles. What about on My Labia?

Right now there's no cosmetic procedure for genital Botox injections. Botox may prove helpful down the road to alleviate various vulvar pain syndromes.

## My Friend Just Had a Vaginoplasty and Is Gushing Over Her New Quim. What's the Deal?

Whatever you call it, "vaginoplasty," "designer vaginoplasty," "vaginal rejuvenation," "revirgination," they are, for the most part, variations on traditional vaginal surgical procedures. When combined with labioplasty (read above), these ops promise to make your vajayjay tighter, narrower, more youthful, and ultrasensitive. While the surgeon is at it, bulges of your bladder, rectum, or vagina can be tucked away, and the hymen can be repaired and remodeled. The goal? To re-create a more "virgin"-like appearance.

Note from Dr. D: Any cosmetic surgery for your V is a personal decision, not a recommendation.

These procedures may be medically indicated in *some* women with vaginal wall relaxation or bulging and hanging genital organs. But plenty of women are pursuing the treatment for the sole purpose of beautification and improved personal and partner sexual satisfaction. Surgery purely for cosmetic reasons and sexual enhancement should be approached intelligently and pursued with an experienced provider.

## My Pubic Area Is Humongous. Can Anything Be Done with It?

Are you talking about the mons pubis, the fleshy mound of fat over your pubic bone? True, the mons pubis can

### G Spot Amplification

Want to enhance your sexual satisfaction? Some women choose to do it by making their G spot bigger. Amplification typically involves an injection of collagen into the anterior wall of the vagina. Warning: There's no scientific information on the safety, efficacy, or long-term satisfaction of this procedure. Your concerns about sexual satisfaction or dysfunction should be further looked into by your gyno or a therapist. So ladies, you're on your own with this one.

get flabby or saggy, particularly with age or weight gain, and some women complain theirs is too bulky and unsightly and can be seen through their bathing suit or gym clothes. Well, there are treatments available, including liposuction and contouring.

## Ever Since I Gave Birth, the Space between My V and Rectum Is Sagging. Is There Anything I Can Do about It?

Yes, there's a procedure called *perineoplasty*, which tightens that area. It promises to lend a more youthful appearance to your vulva and a tighter vaginal opening for enhanced sexual function.

## I've Heard about Vaginal Rejuvenation Spas. Are They Kidding Me?

They kid you not! Spas are popping up all over the place in D.C., N.Y.C., L.A., Palm Beach, Phoenix, even San Miguel, Mexico! These so-called vagina spas promise to turn your already naturally fantastic V into an organ of extraordinary beauty and vitality worthy of a diamond tiara. Special exercises to improve pelvic muscle tone and help with bladder control,

Choosing surgery of *any kind* for these issues requires careful consideration, as does picking a gynecologic or plastic surgeon comfortable and experienced in genital rejuvenation procedures. Make it a priority!

as well as orgasm enhancement, are offered with names like Kegel Phitness, the "Other" Face Lift, and Lip Sync.

Many spas offer a full range of vaginal cosmetic surgery or liposuction techniques. You can get vagina massages or one-on-one vaginal exercise instruction. Or order Linger— an "internal feminine flavoring" treatment that promises to keep your vagina in mint condition. Think of it as an Altoid for your lady parts.

# M

# Menstruation, Moods, and Misery

If men could menstruate ... clearly, menstruation would become an enviable, boast-worthy, masculine event: Men would brag about how long and how much…. Sanitary supplies would be federally funded and free.

—*Gloria Steinem*

Aunt Flow, Cousin Red, that time of the month, the Present or Gift or Visitor, get (one's) redwings, have the painters in, on the rag, red tide, ride the cotton pony, Sally, surf the crimson wave, *that* time of the month, your period…. Listen, whatever you want to call it—you've got it. You're menstruating.

## What Exactly Happens When I Get My Period?

It's this simple: When you menstruate—or get your period—your body sheds the lining of the uterus (womb).

Menstrual blood flows from the uterus through the small opening in your cervix and passes out of your body through the vajayjay. And sometimes it's not so much fun.

## How Long Does a Normal Period Last?

Most menstrual periods last from three to seven days. I'd say that's normal. The average menstrual cycle lasts twenty-eight to thirty days counting from the first day of one period to the first day of the next. Normal cycles can vary from twenty-one to thirty-five days. During an average menstrual cycle, women lose approximately five tablespoons of blood. In general, if you're using more than six to ten pads or tampons a day or soaking through one to two superpads or tampons every hour, let your doctor know. That's probably not normal. If you always wear a yellow polka-dot skirt with a chartreuse-striped halter top every day when you have your period and insist on putting petunias in your hair, I'd say that's probably not normal either. See your mirror.

Q. What did the vampire say to the high school girl?
A. See you next period!

## At What Age Does the Red Tide Usually Start?

Well, it can begin as early as eight years old or as late as sixteen. Most often girls between eleven and twelve years begin their periods for the first time.

FYI: The start of menstruation has its own name: menarche. Sounds French, *oui*? Oh, tell the young *femmes* not to freak if their menstruation cycle is irregular—it takes a while to get into rhythm.

# I Don't Get My Period Every Month, but When It Comes—OMG—It's Impressive. How Weird Is That?

Well, it's not *that* weird. There are reasons, and you should get it checked out. It's common in adolescents and premenopausal women or those with polycystic ovarian syndrome. An abnormal growth in the uterus can lead to "weird" menses. This includes uterine polyps, fibroids (benign muscular tumors), hyperplasia (an overgrowth of uterine tissue and possible cancer precursor), and uterine cancer. Finally, a bleeding disorder that increases bleeding throughout the body such as Von Willebrand's disease or a low platelet count

Q. How did the Red Sea get its name?

A. Cleopatra used to bathe there *periodically.*

## Talking the Talk

Sisters, we know how "special" we feel when we have our periods (ha ha), so maybe that's why menstruation has so many *special* words to define its many manifestations. Here they are:

**Menorrhagia**   heavy or prolonged menstrual bleeding.

**Metrorrhagia**   bleeding in between periods, also known as breakthrough bleeding or spotting.

**Polymenorrhea**   frequent menstrual bleeding, specifically, bleeding that occurs every twenty-one days or less.

**Amenorrhea**   the absence of menses. Primary amenorrhea, when your period hasn't started ever by age sixteen, secondary amenorrhea, when menses are absent for more than three to six months.

**Oligomenorrhea**   fewer than six to eight periods per year.

**Anovulation**   when you don't ovulate. Yay, you say? Well, it can also mean you end up with a heavy period or menses when you do.

IF YOU HAVE *ANY* OF THESE CONDITIONS, SEE YOUR DOCTOR!

can cause a heavy flow. Blood-thinning medications such as Coumadin or aspirin may also cause abnormal periods. Don't mess around—see your doc.

## My Cramps Are No Joke!

Does it help to know you're not alone? Probably not much. But let me tell you: Menstrual cramps of some degree affect more than 50 percent of us, and up to 15 percent of women describe their menstrual cramps as, like, so way severe. Surveys of adolescent girls show that over 90 percent report having menstrual cramps. They can range from mild to quite severe. Mild menstrual cramps may be barely noticeable and of short duration—sometimes it's just a sense of light heaviness in the belly. Severe menstrual cramps can be so painful

Got cramps? Have sex! Orgasms can relieve menstrual cramps in some women.

that they interfere with a woman's regular activities for several days. If this is you—let your doctor know about it. Following are some methods to treat the pain:

- Use a heating pad.
- Think ahead and take NSAIDS (e.g., ibuprofen) a day or so before your period.
- Speak to your gyno about hormonal contraception.
- Get treatment for any underlying condition that's causing cramps.

## Right Before My Period I'm a Bitch on Wheels

And let me guess: Your partner is the pavement. The physical and emotional changes that happen during the days before you get your period are called premenstrual syndrome. PMS affects at least 85 percent of menstruating women, and the symptoms are physical and emotional, but guess what (and don't get annoyed)? The cause is unknown. PMDD, premenstrual dysphoric disorder, is a severe form of PMS that affects a small percentage of women, in which symptoms interfere with work or personal relationships. Does that sound like you? *Get help.* PMS symptoms women experience (as if we have to tell you):

• Emotional: Depression, angry outbursts, irritability, crying spells, anxiety, confusion, social withdrawal, poor concentration, insomnia, increased nap taking, changes in sexual desire.

• Physical: Thirst and appetite changes including food cravings, breast tenderness, bloating and weight gain, headache, swelling of the hands or feet, aches and pains, fatigue, skin problems, gastrointestinal symptoms, abdominal pain.

• Other common conditions: Depression and anxiety, perimenopause, chronic fatigue syndrome, irritable bowel syndrome, and thyroid disease, to name a few, can mimic or overlap with PMS. In addition, certain conditions may worsen right before your period, such as seizure disorders, migraines, asthma, and allergies.

## Is There Any Way I Can Stop Feeling So Crazy?

Absolutely!

• Try regular aerobic exercise, relaxation through yoga, meditation, breathing exercises, and getting enough sleep.

## The Ten Definitive Signs of PMS

1. Everyone around you has an attitude problem.

2. You're adding chocolate chips to your cheese omelet.

3. The dryer has shrunk every last pair of your jeans.

4. Your partner is suddenly agreeing to everything you say.

5. You're using your cell phone to dial up every bumper sticker that says, "How's my driving? Call 1-800-###-####."

6. Everyone's head looks like an invitation to batting practice.

7. You're convinced there's a God and he's male.

8. You're counting the days until menopause.

9. You're sure that everyone's scheming to drive you crazy.

10. The ibuprofen bottle is empty, and you bought it yesterday.

• Make some diet changes. Dishes rich in complex carbohydrates can reduce mood symptoms *and* food cravings. Avoiding caffeine and alcohol may help—but so may that glass of wine. Less fat, salt, and sugar and eating small frequent meals is also a good idea.

• Use supplements. Calcium, 1,200 mg a day, can reduce PMS symptoms. Magnesium may help reduce water retention, breast tenderness, and mood symptoms. The B vitamins, especially when you get them from your diet, can also help.

• Check with your doctor about prescription meds. For those who are really going off the PMS deep end, hormonal contraceptives like the pill may lessen the physical symptoms of PMS. Low-dose diuretics, or water pills, can help with water retention. Finally, certain antidepressants can be used, typically during days fourteen to twenty-eight of the cycle or every day if need be. Anti-anxiety pills may also be right for some sisters.

For more information on how prescription meds can help with issues like perimenopause and menopause, see "Hormones, Hot Flashes, and Jalapeño Peppers" (page 78).

## The Scoop on Sanitary Products

**PADS**    Pads come in different sizes, styles, and thicknesses. Some have wings that fold under your underwear for better protection. Some are fragrant; avoid these if they irritate your skin.

**PANTY LINERS**    Liners are thinner and shorter for lighter flow and come in various shapes and sizes including those meant for thongs.

**TAMPONS**    Tampons are available in a variety of sizes depending on flow, fragrant or non, and with or without an applicator. They should not be left in for more than eight hours and usually need to be changed more frequently. Tampons can be worn while swimming and exercising without a problem.

Disposable sanitary napkins appeared in Germany as early as the 1880s but were unavailable to American women because of the Comstock Laws (part of a campaign for legislating public morality in the United States).

**MENSTRUAL CUP**    This nonabsorbent reusable cup is inserted in the vagina and collects menstrual flow. It can be worn for up to twelve hours and eliminates the need for other sanitary products.

**REUSABLE MENSTRUAL PADS**    For the environmentally obsessed who don't mind really being "on the rag."

# N

# Nutritional Know-Hows and No-No's

Q. Does female vaginal fluid have *any* nutritional value?

A. The short answer: There are no benefits or nutritional value in female or male ejaculate. The slightly longer short answer is that thanks to the extremely low nutritional values, vaginal fluids are an excellent addition to a calorie-controlled diet.

## You Know the Old Saying You Are What You Eat? What Should I Eat to Keep My Vag Sweet and Healthy?

The answer is *not* sugar, honey. The fact is any diet that's healthy for your entire body will benefit your V. Foods high in sugar have a tendency to increase the risk of yeast infections. So avoid processed foods, baked goods, alcohol, and sweet drinks for the same reason. But if your vagina isn't happy and getting the balance of vitamins and minerals it needs, you could be more prone to irritation and infection. Here are some foods that will help keep you sweet and healthy:

- Yogurt—a key ingredient, acidophilus, is a huge help in preventing and treating yeast infections. You can also take acidophilus supplements.
- Fruits, vegetables, and whole grains—which promote overall good health.
- Cranberry juice or taking cranberry tablets— decreases urinary tract infection.

## My Gynecologist Told Me to Take Calcium and Vitamin D, But I'm Not Clear Why

First of all, sister, if you don't understand something your doc tells you, ask questions. Vitamin D and calcium are usually suggested for bone health, so it makes sense that you're confused. But these supplements have other benefits, too. The Institute of Medicine, which is an independent, nonprofit organization, recommends for overall good health a total daily calcium intake of 1,300 mg for girls ages nine to eighteen, 1,000 mg for women ages nineteen to fifty, and 1,200 mg for women fifty-one and older. As we said before, if you want a healthy vagina, you need a healthy body. While it's best to get your calcium in foods such as dairy, broccoli, almonds, and salmon, supplements may also be needed. Calcium supplements should be taken in divided doses.

Don't eat anything your great-great grandmother wouldn't recognize as food. There are a great many foodlike items in the supermarket your ancestors wouldn't recognize as food.
—*Michael Pollan*

Don't take it all at once because your body will have an easier time absorbing it. But don't overdo it! Too much calcium can lead to kidney stones or heart disease. FYI: You need Vitamin D to absorb the calcium. Fortified dairy products provide dietary D, but the main source is sunlight.

Alert! Eating disorders such as anorexia and bulimia can cause menstrual irregularity or even amenorrhea. And prolonged amenorrhea is linked to bone loss.

Since most of us slather ourselves with sunscreen—and you should—supplemental vitamin D of 1,000 IUs a day or less is a safe alternative.

## Are There Any Natural Herbs That Can Give My Sex Drive a Boost?

There are no guarantees, but you can try arginine, which is an amino acid found in granola, oatmeal, nuts, seeds, eggs, coconut milk, and root veggies. Or you can get it in a supplement form. It *claims* to increase blood flow to the genitals and enhance sex drive.

## What about Aphrodisiacs?

CHOCOLATE   Chocolate contains phenylethylamine and serotonin, chemicals that promote a feeling of well-being.

RED WINE   Red wine is relaxing and contains resveratrol, an antioxidant that helps boost blood flow and improve circulation.

OYSTERS   Oysters contain zinc, which enhances sexual potency in men, and omega-3 fatty acids, which improve nervous system function.

**BANANAS** Bananas have a suggestive phallic shape and contain potassium.

**AVOCADO** Avocados have a phallic "testicular" shape; their vitamin E content is helpful in hormonal production and thus sexual response.

**SALMON AND WALNUTS** Both these foods contain omega-3 fatty acids needed for sex hormone production.

**CHILE PEPPERS** Chilies contain capsaicin and cause sweating, increased heart rate, and circulation, even in the genitals.

**FIGS** Figs are sexually suggestive based on appearance, since an open fig looks similar to the female sex organs.

**HONEY** Honey is rich in B vitamins and boron, needed for sex hormone production.

**SOY** Soy in the diet and in supplement form contains isoflavones, which promote vaginal lubrication because of their estrogenlike qualities (not appropriate for women with breast cancer).

# I'm Pregnant. Should I Take Special Vitamins?

Prenatal vitamins are recommended for most women during pregnancy to obtain the extra recommended daily intake of calcium, iron, and folic acid. Here's why:

- Folic acid (folate) lowers the risk of neural tube defects such as spina bifida.
- Iron will help prevent anemia, or low blood count.
- DHA, omega-3 fatty acids, found in many fish, helps promote a healthy nervous system.

Keep in mind that excess amounts of some vitamins or minerals, and many herbal supplements, can be harmful during pregnancy. Speak with your doc before taking *any*.

## What About Gaining Weight While I'm Pregnant?

Well, you don't want to go overboard, but you should definitely pack on some pounds. Most moms-to-be who are already a healthy weight should gain between twenty-five and thirty-five pounds during pregnancy. An additional three hundred calories a day is a good rule, and small frequent meals rather than three large ones are often best. But like most things in life, it's best not to overdo it. Keep in mind: *Packing on too many pounds increases the risk for gestational diabetes and/or very big babies, which means a tough delivery and the possibility of more extensive V trauma.*

> Good sex is like a good bridge game. If you don't have a good partner, you'd better have a good hand.
> —*Mae West*

# O

# The Big O! Oh! O! Oh! Ahhh ... and All Things Orgasmic and Otherwise

Electric flesh-arrows traversing the body; a rainbow of color strikes the eyelids. A foam of music falls over the ears. It is the gong of the orgasm.

*—Anaïs Nin*

Sure—like this is news: *Unlike guys, we need to be in the mood to have sex.* If we're stressed, pissed off, feeling fat or unattractive, slightly short of smelling like a rose or not totally groomed, thinking about the laundry, angsting over our kids, worried about work, down and blue, freaked out about exams, exhausted, achy, not feeling safe, or dealing with money woes, the chances we're going to feel like hot babes and have an orgasm are as likely as Lady Gaga joining a nunnery. Plus, there are plenty of women who are using different ways to get physical and emotional comfort without intercourse or orgasm. So even though some of us can take an orgasm or leave it, and other sisters may be in it just to please their partners, for the rest of us, we want and need the Big O, and we'll do *whatever* to have one. Wait! Make that two or three.

## What's Happening to My Body While I'm Coming?

We call the desire to have sex the *libido*. Your libido can suddenly be charged up for no apparent reason, or because your partner is making you hot, or because other thoughts or images are turning you on.

Arousal, on the other hand, is the result of sexual stimulation *plus* desire. Your body knows it: Your blood pressure, heart rate, breathing rate, and body temperature all rise. Your nips are erect, and your labia and clit are engorged with blood and are supersensitive. Your cha-cha is juicy and expands. It's sayin' "come and get me." Well, hold on … you're *almost* there. Contractions of the genital muscles and then … and then … an overwhelming feeling of release! Now, that was intense.

One of the big shocks of the twentieth century was that our nation's sex symbol, Marilyn Monroe, claimed she never achieved orgasm by any of her famous lovers, like John F. Kennedy, Frank Sinatra, Joe DiMaggio, and Arthur Miller.

## I Used to Love Sex and Was the Queen of O. Now It Takes Forever, or It Doesn't Happen at All, and Truthiness? I Couldn't Care Less.

It probably doesn't make you feel any better to know that problems in this department aren't uncommon. And there usually isn't just one reason keeping you from wanting to have sex or reaching a climax. Best advice? Be open about it and speak with your gyno. I can promise this issue is raised over and over again. Join in the discussion.

Meanwhile, here are a few possibilities:

**GETTING OLDER**  You might still look as hot as Jennifer Lopez, but your libido doesn't know; it slows down while the years add up. Usually this is NOT a five-alarmer unless it's interfering with your relationship. Declining estrogen and androgens (male hormones) because of aging, or natural or surgical menopause, may lessen your desire for sex.

Some women scream, some women moan, some women whimper, some women LOL, some women weep, some women thank god, some women recite Emily Dickinson, some women curse, some women stay silent.

**MEDICATIONS**  Occasionally medications such as birth control pills, SSRI antidepressants, and beta-blockers used to treat high blood pressure can alter libido.

**MEDICAL ISSUES**  Coronary artery disease, arthritis, cancer, diabetes, and other conditions may affect your sex drive. Depression is a common cause of decreased libido. In fact, sometimes, it's hard to know whether decreased desire is because you're feeling down—or taking medications to beat it—or a combo of both. Total bummer.

**BODY IMAGE**  Body image plays a huge role in sexual desire. Sisters who feel unattractive, overweight, or out of shape are more likely to avoid sex altogether.

**RELATIONSHIP PROBLEMS**  Can definitely put a damper on sex. That's why desire is so much more intense and sex is more frequent when you're with a new partner.

Libido can become dulled and sex less frequent in long-term relationships. This is a problem only if you or your partner is unhappy about

Too Bad: Medications prescribed for men like Viagra and Cialis have not been put on the list for women ... *yet.*

having less nookie. But if you can't get turned on because you resent your partner, well, that's another story.

## Dealing with It

Hey, so if you want to hop back in the saddle, you've got to discover and then deal with the underlying issues.

- Set up a time to sit down and talk to your partner about it.
- Diet, exercise, and a healthy lifestyle are key.
- Stress reduction and adequate sleep are essential.
- Set aside time for intimacy without other distractions. Shut off the television, computer, and mobile phone; be sure the kids are asleep or your roommate isn't going to walk in.
- Consider OTC supplements, although effectiveness is varied. Avlimil is an OTC herbal tablet promising increased desire and pleasure. Zestra, which is botanical massage oil, can be applied to the clitoris, labia, and vagina, and also claims to increase arousal. DHEA is an OTC nutritional supplement and a chemical precursor to testosterone. WARNING: *None* of these products have been proven effective or safe, or are FDA approved.
- Try testosterone therapy, which is available by prescription. It uses a "male" hormone (an androgen), which is also produced in small amounts by a woman's adrenal glands and ovaries. The treatment has been proven to improve female sexual function and is often used "off label." But check this out: There are side effects to consider, including deepening of the voice, acne, hair growth in typically male places (upper lip, chin), enlarged clitoris, and alteration in lipid profile. Note that testosterone is not approved by the U.S. Food and Drug Administration for treating sexual problems in women.

**SMOKING, ALCOHOL, DRUGS** These can definitely lower your sex drive and response. Smoking in particular decreases the blood flow to the genitals and can cause issues with arousal. Ladies, another reason to quit!

## Wanna Have an Orgasm? Well ...

Memory is like an orgasm. It's a lot better if you don't have to fake it.

—Anonymous

It's not always about the penis. Some of us won't have an orgasm with vaginal intercourse but can come with manual clitoral stimulation from a partner, a vibrator, or masturbation. There's an FDA-approved clitoral suction device, EROS, which may improve arousal and orgasm by boosting clitoral blood flow. There are also lots of vibrators on the market that are much less expensive and can definitely do the trick.

## It's Just Not Happening and I'm Miserable. I Tried Practically Everything. What Else Can I Do?

Orgasm can cause bad breath! Doctors have detected a slight odor on the tongues of women for up to an hour after they've had intercourse. Note to self: Keep some gum or mints on the nightstand.

Has anyone spoken to you about sex therapy? You go either alone or with your partner to a highly trained physician, psychologist, or social worker. Usually the therapy session will include education about the normal sexual response, as well as ways to deal with cultural, religious, and other personal sexual concerns. Sex therapists work to improve communication between partners. They use visual aids, devices, and give "homework." Therapy may help partners agree on sexual

## Faking It

Well, lots of my patients fake it and admit to it, and it's no big deal. In fact, as many as two-thirds of women admit to faking orgasms at some point in their lives—and it's not just during vaginal intercourse. Women also say they've pretended to orgasm during oral and phone sex. Remember *When Harry Met Sally*?

Although there may be a twinge of guilt, we have our reasons: You want to please your partner, you feel "sorry" for your partner and don't want to cause any embarrassment or feelings of inadequacy, or you just want to get it over with so you can get some sleep. As long as a woman CAN have an orgasm, it's no biggie if there's no O every time she makes love. Sometimes a gal's gotta do what a gal's gotta do.

practices and frequency. Visit www.aasect.org for further information.

Note: Ladies with prior sexual, emotional, or physical abuse could benefit from collaboration with a trained mental health professional. Those with underlying medical conditions causing sexual problems would benefit from appropriate physician referral as well. A team approach is best in these cases.

# P

## Pap Smear, Papilloma Virus, and Protection for All Lovely Lady Flowers

*Ross (picks up a surgical instrument):* Quack. Quack. Quack. Quack. Quack.
*Carol:* Ross ... that opens my cervix.

—Friends

Maybe this isn't the sexiest info you'll ever read. Okay. So, it's no Kama Sutra. Still, getting a grip on what's going on in your cervix can be a real lifesaver. Peeps! Please! Pay! Attention!

### The Primer

Your cervix is made up of several layers of cells. The outer layer is composed of "squamous" cells. The opening is made of glandular cells. These two kinds of cells meet in a place called the "transition zone" (T-zone). It may sound romantic, but it's really a danger zone because the T-zone is the most common place where abnormal cells can be found.

It's a good idea to avoid *anything* in your vagina a couple of days before your Pap—that means spermicide, lubricant, tampons, and ... A finger, penis, dildo, etc.

And that's where the Pap smear comes in: It screens for cancer of the cervix. Traditionally the Pap smear involves a sampling of cells from your cervix with a brush or spatula wielded by your gyno. Your doc will need to use a speculum; the procedure is a little uncomfy, but not painful.

You don't need to get a Pap smear before you're twenty-one years old, and for lots of women older than that, depending on your risk, you can get it done every one to three years. If you've had a hysterectomy with your cervix removed for benign reasons, you also won't need one. Many women over sixty-five can stop hav-

Yo mama's so stupid, she went to Dr. Dre for a Pap smear.

ing Pap smears in many cases unless you're involved with a new sex partner or multiple partners.

If you receive news your Pap smear is "abnormal," consult with your health care practitioner about your diagnosis and treatment options.

## My Doctor Told Me I Have HPV. What's Going On?

Unfortunately, these days I'm giving out the same news pretty often. There are more than one hundred different strains of HPV, and not all of them cause cancer, so it's hard to say exactly what's happening in *your* case. "Low risk strains" cause *only* genital warts. "High-risk strains" are linked to cancer of the anus, cervix, vulva, vagina, penis, head, and neck. While close to 80 percent of women are exposed to HPV in their lifetime, the vast majority won't develop cancer as the immune system deals with the HPV virus before it causes cancer. Other HPV facts to know:

- For some, HPV is persistent and can lead to precancer and then cancer.
- HPV is spread by direct skin-to-skin contact, including sexual intercourse, oral sex, anal sex, and hand-to-genital contact.
- Most with HPV have no symptoms.
- Most HPV infections are temporary and resolve within two years.
- Some HPV infections persist.
- Certain high-risk strains of HPV may be tested for alone or in combination with a Pap smear to screen for cervix cancer.
- HPV screening is not recommended for women under thirty years old.

## So, Who Needs a Pap ... and *When?*

- Women younger than thirty should have a Pap at least every two years.
- Women thirty and older should have a Pap at least every two years. After three normal Paps in a row, a woman in this age group may have a Pap every three years if she doesn't have a history of moderate or severe dysplasia (precancer cells that are significantly abnormal), if she's not infected with HIV, and if her immune system isn't weakened, and if she wasn't exposed to diethylstilbestrol (DES) before birth.
- Women older than thirty may have an HPV test at the same time as a Pap test. If the results of both tests are normal, these women do not need another Pap or HPV for two to three years.

# What about the HPV Vaccine—Does It Work?

We know. We know. You've heard a lot of negative talk about the vaccine. But the most common side effect is just tenderness at the injection site. And it can prevent HPV, the most common sexually transmitted infection.

There are two available optional vaccines to protect against HPV. Both are given in three doses over a six-month period. Neither will protect against all types of HPV. Here are some important facts about the vaccine:

> When I told my 13-year-old daughter Alice I was taking her to get a vaccine that could help prevent cancer, she was mildly intrigued. "Cool," she allowed, "but I hate shots."
>
> —*Claudia Wallis*, Newsweek

- Vaccines are recommended for girls ages nine to twenty-six years.
- Vaccines are best given *before* a woman is sexually active and is exposed to HPV. However, young women can receive the vaccine even if they've already had sex, had genital warts, received abnormal Pap test results, or been infected with HPV.
- If a woman is already infected with one type of HPV, the vaccines will not protect against disease caused by that type.
- Vaccines are not a treatment for current HPV infection.
- Vaccines are not recommended for pregnant women.
- Women who are vaccinated should still have regular Pap tests.
- The most common side effect is soreness in the arm where the shot is given and, rarely, headache, fatigue, nausea, dizziness, and/or fainting.

# Should *Everyone* Get a Colposcopy?

Hardly! A *colposcopy* is a test that offers a magnified view of your cervix and V. Your gyno may recommend one if your Pap or HPV test is abnormal, or if you have warts on your cervix, an inflamed cervix (cervicitis), cervical polyps, pain, or bleeding. It's done in the office, takes around five to ten minutes, and is just a little uncomfortable. For at least a day *before* the test, you should avoid douching, tampons, vaginal meds, and sex. It's also a good idea to schedule this test when you're not having a heavy day of menstrual bleeding. Avoid anything in your V for a few days *after* the procedure and give your doc a holler *immediately* if you experience heavy vaginal bleeding, severe lower abdominal pain, fever, or chills. Depending on the results, you may need to be checked more often or you may need further testing or treatment.

# What If My Test Is Weird?

You mean abnormal? Well, several treatments are available. Sisters with mild cervical abnormalities, particularly if they're not thirty years old yet, can have their condition monitored with more frequent Paps and colposcopies. Lots of times, it gets better by itself without any treatment. If that's not your case, abnormal cells can be frozen, or removed via laser (LEEP) or surgically (cone biopsy).

Yo! There's an excellent chance you can prevent cervical cancer by having regular Pap tests!

LEEP (loop electrosurgical excision procedure) is an office procedure, done with local anesthesia, in which a thin wire loop, charged with electric current, removes a cone-shaped area of the cervix.

## Cervical Cancer

Cervical cancer affects an estimated twelve thousand American women each year. About half the cases are in women who have never had a Pap test. The good news: In most cases, cervical cancer can be cured if it's found and treated early. It usually occurs in women older than forty, but anyone can get it. Risk factors include multiple sexual partners, having a male partner who has multiple sex partners, early age at first intercourse (younger than eighteen), smoking, family history of cervical cancer, immunosuppressant, and in utero exposure to DES (a medicine used from 1940 to 1971 to prevent miscarriage). Symptoms can include abnormal bleeding or watery vaginal discharge.

FYI: Many women have no symptoms. Diagnosis is often suspected with Pap and confirmed with cervical biopsy. After diagnosis, the extent of disease is determined with a pelvic exam and various imaging tests of the bladder, rectum, and pelvis. Treatment of cervical cancer depends on how advanced it is, but it can involve LEEP or cone biopsy, simple or more complex hysterectomy, chemotherapy and radiation.

Cone biopsy is done in an operating room with anesthesia to remove a cone-shaped portion of the cervix, particularly in cases where cervical cancer is suspected. This procedure allows for removal and evaluation of tissue to confirm the degree of abnormality and to be sure the abnormal area is removed completely.

Complications after LEEP or cone biopsy include bleeding, infection, or weakening of the cervix in future pregnancy. Follow-up testing and treatment depends on results and circumstances.

# Q

## Quandaries, Predicaments, Snafus, and the Complexities of Quims

Sisters, sometimes the vagina lets us down. Try as we do to keep it happy, there are conditions that perplex, vex, puzzle, mystify, bewilder, flummox, stupefy, dumbfound, and, alas, make us blue. It's not pretty. That doesn't mean there aren't explanations and answers, but they may not solve the problem forever or make us happy. In this chapter, we'll look at some of these situations. Just know that whatever you're going through, I've seen it before—you're not alone. And remember: *Nothing is too gross to talk about.*

## Bartholin's Cyst/Abscess

The Bartholin's glands are located at the opening of your V. If you're into exact locations, imagine your vajayjay is a clock and the gland ducts are located at the four and eight o'clock positions. If the opening of your gland becomes blocked with mucus, a cyst can develop. Don't freak out if this happens; it's not uncommon. Bartholin's cysts are collections of fluid usually between the size of a pea and a golf ball and can cause pain during sex or even when you're just walking or sitting. Obviously, it's no fun. If you're uncomfortable, then your gyno will probably suggest draining the cyst. If the cyst gets infected and becomes a Bartholin's abscess, you'll know it because it *really* hurts and draining will definitely be in order. Once it's drained of pus, the pain leaves immediately. The good news is that sometimes draining happens spontaneously just while taking sitz baths or warm soaks. If not, you may need to have it done surgically. Antibiotics and pain medication may be prescribed.

Bummer Alert: History can repeat itself.

## Vulvar Abscess

This usually starts out as simple infection in the vulvar skin. What causes it? Well, risk factors include obesity, poor hygiene, and shaving or waxing. Sometimes a vulvar abscess will develop because your immune system isn't working well enough to fight infections. If your doc finds a tender, red, swollen, and painful collection of pus on your vulva, a diagnosis of a vulvar abscess will probably be made. Treatment includes antibiotics, drainage, warm soaks, and a follow-up to be sure the infection doesn't travel beneath the skin level.

Bummer Alert: It can happen again.

# Vaginal Polyps and Cysts

Polyps are fleshy growths that are typically benign and won't need any treatment (yay!) *unless* they are growing,

Vaginal cysts can form in infancy.

are painful, or cause bleeding. Cysts form when a gland or duct is clogged and liquid collects in a sac. These can occur inside the vagina. Treatment is not needed unless they're getting bigger or making you uncomfortable.

# Vulvar Skin Tags

These are outgrowths of normal skin and look like tiny flags on narrow stalks. They're more common as we age and often happen on the site of friction, including your groin and vulva. Tags can stand alone or have many friends. In this instance, we'd prefer loners. Your doc won't bother doing anything about a skin tag unless it's irritating you or growing. But lots of women want them removed for cosmetic reasons. You can get them taken off at your doctor's office. Only local anesthesia is required.

Bummer Alert: Did someone say "déjà vu"?

# Sebaceous Cysts

Sebaceous cysts are dome-shaped, soft, smooth white bumps under the surface of your vulva's skin. To be more specific, they are closed sacs that contain keratin, a "pasty" or "cheesy" protein. They're usually smaller than a pea and painless. There can be a single one standing on its own or several. A diagnosis is usually made by your doc just by looking, and treatment is optional.

# Inguinal Lymph Nodes

We all have lymph nodes in our groin, and normal ones are usually less than one centimeter in diameter and they're usually soft. If you're thin, you might be able to feel them. But there are instances when these friendly nodes become inflamed, enlarged, and tender. It might be the result of infection or trauma, for example, because of an infection from shaving. Less commonly, cancer or other illness can be the cause. So it's a good idea to see your doctor if your nodes are persistently enlarged.

# Vaginal Cancer

This is somewhat rare—only about 3 percent of genital cancers start in the vagina, but other cancers can metastasize there. Primary vaginal cancer is more common in women with multiple lifetime sexual partners, intercourse at an early age, smoking, and HPV. The most common symptom is abnormal bleeding. Your health care provider will take a biopsy, and if it's positive, various treatments will be considered.

# Imperforate Hymen

As if you don't know, the hymen is a thin membrane that surrounds the vaginal opening. The most common shape is usually a half-moon. Sorry gals, no metaphorical stars—that is, until it's "broken" by your first intercourse, tampon use, or trauma. Sometimes, the hymen is too thick or incompletely "broken," and it obstructs the vaginal opening. How would you know? Well, typically,

## Congenital Absence of Vagina

Vaginal agenesis, or Mayer-Rokitansky-Kuster-Hauser (MRKH) syndrome, refers to the congenital absence of the vagina. In other words, you're born without a vagina. This is relatively uncommon; approximately one in four thousand to ten thousand women are affected. Ovaries are present and functional, and the uterus and cervix may be present, but menstruation never happens, and women can't have intercourse. Diagnosis is made with history, physical exam, and imaging. Treatment involves the use of vaginal dilators to gradually create a vagina suitable for intercourse. In some cases, surgery is used to create a vagina.

a young woman will be unable to insert a tampon or have sex because "there's a blockage." Diagnosis is usually made by physical exam, and treatment involves simple surgical repair.

# Vaginal Septum

This is a thick band of either horizontal or vertical tissue that may shorten or misshape the inside of your V, and it's a problem you're born with. Some women with a vaginal septum complain of difficulty inserting tampons, bleeding even though a tampon is inserted, and painful sex. On the other hand, some have no symptoms. Diagnosis is made by exam, and treatment, if needed, is surgical.

# R

# Rectum ... Nearly Killed 'Em

> Just like the four main directions (North, South, East and West) the body also possesses four openings or doors—the East door is Mouth, the West door is Rectum, the North door is Head, while the South door is Private part.
>
> —*Atharva Veda*

Are we as simple as a compass? Well, not for most Western women. About three-quarters of the population (this estimate is *not* based on research!) feels squeamish when it comes to talking about rectal and anal issues. Even my smartest, most daring friends get all uptight and coy about their backside. But I say, "Hey, Girlfriend, what's the big deal? The rectum is just another part of your anatomy. Why play favorites?" And then I explain anal issues without coating anything with sugar. Okay, so that might be a bad cliché!

We're not all assholes, but we all have one.

The rectum is the lower part of your large intestine where your body stores stool. The anus is the opening of the rectum through which stool passes out of your body. Problems with the rectum and anus are common. They include hemorrhoids, abscesses, incontinence, and cancer of the rectum or anus. If you have *any* anal or rectal troubles—especially if you have pain or bleeding—don't be too embarrassed to speak with your doctor about it.

Buzz Kill: The bottom wall of the vagina is the same as the top wall of the rectum. That's why injury to one can lead to injury to the other. Rectal problems or infections can directly lead to vaginal infections.

## It Feels Like There's an Itchy Lump in My Rectum. Uhhh ... What's Going on in There?

It's probably no biggie—although it might be large. The most likely diagnosis is *hemorrhoids*, which are nothing more than enlarged or swollen veins in your rectum. Often they can be felt, or seen, around the outside of your anus, or they may be hidden inside. There might be other less-than-charming symptoms such as rectal bleeding, pain, bulging tissue around the anus, leakage of feces, or difficulty cleaning after a bowel movement. Even though there's no reason to be ashamed, this might not be something you want to talk about on a first date.

Hemorrhoids may develop because you're overweight, pregnant, standing, or sitting for long periods, or straining during physical labor or constipation.

**Testing**  Diagnosis is made by clinical exam or by an anoscopy (looking inside the anus with a small instrument).

### Treatment

- Prevention of constipation and avoiding straining during a bowel movement.
- Sitz baths for fifteen minutes, two or three times a day, give relief. These are warm-water soaks that improve blood flow and relax the muscle around the anus.
- Topical creams or suppositories available OTC or by prescription for relief of pain, itching, and swelling.
- Banding, cautery, or surgical therapy for larger hemorrhoids.

## After a Bowel Movement I Feel a Burning or Tearing and Then a Throbbing Pain That Lasts for a Few Minutes ... Sometimes Even Longer

You could be suffering from *fissures*, which are tears in the lining of the anus. It's usually not a big deal, and the fissure can heal spontaneously. If not, no worries, there are treatments. But if you're freaking out, it's understandable. Even a small amount of blood in the toilet bowl can be frightening. Anal fissures are caused by trauma including passage of bulky hard stools. Or they might be related to intestinal conditions such as Crohn's Disease. Speak with your doctor.

## Treatment

- Eliminating constipation with fiber and laxatives.
- Softening your stools with OTC stool softeners.
- Sitz baths.
- Using nitroglycerin ointment or Botox injections.
- Seeing a specialist for surgical treatment.

## I Love My Baby, and I Would've Done *Anything* to Give Birth to Her, Including Having My Rectum Ripped Apart—Which Actually Happened! What Gives?

We bet she's the most beautiful little one in the world. That said, you may have had an *obstetrical tear* involving the anal sphincter and rectum. Tears can lead to chronic conditions including anorectal abscess, fecal incontinence, and painful sex. There are certain circumstances that put women at higher risk for the condition, including delivery of a big baby, Indian or Asian ethnicity, first pregnancy, episiotomy, length of labor, and operative delivery with forceps or vacuum.

## Treatment

- Time and patience while healing during your postpartum period.
- Sitz baths.
- Stool softeners to avoid constipation and straining.
- Topical and oral analgesics for pain.

- In months following delivery, estrogen cream and lubrication may help with painful sex.
- Surgical consultation or procedure may be needed for more chronic issues.

## How Can I Say This? I'm Sooo Itchy!

*Anal pruritus*, or anal itching, is annoying but usually just a benign condition and nothing to lose sleep about. Dietary factors and fecal soilage are the most common causes, but overzealous cleansing, hemorrhoids, fissures, skin conditions like psoriasis, or cancer could also contribute to this condition. Interestingly, itching is often made worse by application of multiple medications and products for relief. In this instance, the adage "less is more" might be the way to go.

> Take it easy doc. You're boldly going where no man has dared to go.
> —Dave Barry, on his colonoscopy

**Testing** Diagnosis is usually made with a good history, clinical exam, and in some cases a skin biopsy or sigmoidoscopy or colonoscopy.

**Treatment** Treatment is aimed at finding and eliminating the cause:
- Avoid trigger foods such as coffee, tea, cola, chocolate, tomatoes, and citrus.
- Use nonperfumed laundry detergent and mild bath products.
- Nix baby wipes, which may contain alcohol or witch hazel and can worsen symptoms.

Also:

- Wipe with premoistened toilet paper.
- Try 1 percent hydrocortisone cream twice daily to the anus.
- Apply protective ointments containing zinc oxide topically.
- Take antihistamines until local treatments start to work.

## I Notice Blood in the Toilet After I Have a Bowel Movement. Is It Serious?

*Rectal bleeding* is common but should always be checked out by your doctor. It's most often caused by hemorrhoids or an anal fissure (we've already talked about those), but

### The Colonoscopy

A *colonoscopy* allows a medical expert to view the lining of your rectum and the entire colon. It's an all-in-one procedure used to screen for colon cancer and to evaluate rectal bleeding, unexplained iron deficiency anemia, or chronic abdominal or rectal pain. Preparing for it isn't the most fun thing in the world. It's certainly not the time to plan a night out on the town. In fact, it's probably a good idea to make your toilet your best friend because a bowel prep, or complete cleansing of the colon with a liquid medication and laxatives, is needed prior to colonoscopy. Right before your colonoscopy, you'll be sedated with IV medication. And then you wake up! And it's over! Most patients recover easily after colonoscopy, and complications are rare. Every grown-up beginning at age fifty or earlier should undergo colon cancer screening, even if you don't have any symptoms. Barium enema and stool tests are also used to evaluate rectal problems. Fun!

other causes include colon or rectal cancer, colon polyps, colitis, and diverticulosis.

**Testing**  The best test for rectal bleeding depends on your age, symptoms, and history. A rectal exam may be all that's needed for diagnosis. Anoscopy is done in the office and allows inspection of the anus and lower rectum. Sigmoidoscopy examines the rectum and most of the lower colon. It's also done without sedation in the office.

**Treatment**  Treatment of rectal bleeding depends on its underlying cause. In some cases, no treatment is needed, and reassurance can be provided.

## I Enjoy Anal Sex. Is There Anything I Should Be Worried About?

On the upside, anal sex cannot cause pregnancy. On the downside, it can cause tiny tears in the anus. That's why some sexually transmitted diseases can be transmitted during anal sex including HIV, herpes, and HPV. Lubrication is highly recommended during anal sex to avoid tears or trauma. So if you take care, you can just enjoy yourself.

## For the Last Few Months My Bowel Movements Have Been Irregular. Is There Something I Can Do about It?

There's an obsession with bowel function throughout the world, and Americans are no exception. But the truth is, one size does not fit all. How many times you drop a load varies widely from several bowel movements a day to one every two or three days. Generally, you're considered constipated if a bowel movement hasn't occurred for three or more days. That said, let's *move* on.

**IRREGULARITY** Irregularity can occur during pregnancy, menstruation, and menopause. Symptoms include constipation, diarrhea, gas, irritable bowel, and discomfort. Don't worry. Most of these conditions aren't serious and can be easily managed with diet changes and judicial use of OTC medications. Rarely are chronic symptoms the sign of a more serious condition.

**CONSTIPATION** Constipation involves hard or infrequent stools that may be painful. In most cases, constipation is not a sign of a serious problem. A high-fiber diet, plenty of water, exercising, and not holding your stool will prevent constipation. A laxative may be recommended if constipation persists; keep in mind that overuse of stimulant laxatives may cause bowel dependency.

**DIARRHEA** Diarrhea is having three or more loose bowel movements per day and may involve cramping. Although it can be uncomfortable, it's generally not a serious condition. Certain foods as well as medical conditions can cause the problem. You should contact your doctor if diarrhea lasts longer than twenty-four hours, is bloody or associated with fever, since you may have an infection or other problem requiring more aggressive workup and treatment.

**IRRITABLE BOWEL SYNDROME (IBS)** IBS mainly affects women ages thirty to fifty, and symptoms can be intermittent. The cause is unclear, but the colon seems to be more sensitive in general. Symptoms include abdominal pain, gas, bloating, alternating constipation and diarrhea, and mucus in the stool. You should see your doctor for

## Simple Ways to Prevent Anorectal Problems

- Eat a high-fiber diet. It's one of the best ways to soften your stools. Fiber is found in fruits and vegetables or can be taken as an OTC supplement. Twenty to thirty-five grams of dietary fiber are recommended daily.
- Keep the area clean and dry.
- Use nonperfumed soap and unscented toilet paper.
- Avoid feminine sprays or talc.
- Sleep in loose-fitting garments.
- Nix tight thongs.
- Use a bidet.
- Wipe with toilet paper moistened with water or an OTC hygienic cleansing solution such as Balneol.

any persistent symptoms to ensure you don't have a more serious condition.

**GAS**   Gas is embarrassing (unless you're into fart jokes). It affects those who are lactose intolerant and those who have trouble digesting beans and certain vegetables such as cabbage and broccoli. You can prevent gas by eliminating dietary triggers or taking an OTC treatment to reduce gas.

# S

## *Sex and Consequences: Sex You Won't Forget (But Wish You Could)...*

Even though a lot of people already have one, it's not like the latest iPod. This isn't something you want. Sexually transmitted infections (STIs), which are also known as sexually transmitted diseases (STDs), are spread person-to-person through intimate contact. STIs aren't picky; they'll infect women (and men) of all ages and backgrounds. And they shouldn't be ignored like annoying spam. Respond to them. If the infection isn't treated, some STIs can cause permanent damage, such as infertility, cancer, and even death (in the case of HIV/AIDS). STIs can spread easily because you may not know your sex partner is infected. In fact, some people with an STI who don't know it pass it along without realizing they're infected. Talk about buzz kill.

# Which Are the Most Common Infections? And How Can I Tell If I Have One?

Just like guys, there are plenty of ways to pick up an STI and lots of different kinds you can get.

## Gonorrhea and Chlamydia

Even a girlfriend who could win the I Spy championship hands down can have gonorrhea and chlamydia and not have a clue. That's why half of women who have it don't know it. "Luckier" women experience vaginal itching, abnormal vaginal discharge, painful sex, irregular vaginal bleeding, or burning with urination. Both these infections spread during sexual intercourse, and anal and oral sex. And you don't need semen to spread the infections. On the upside, you can't catch these STIs on inanimate objects like the toilet seat. On the downside, these infections are repeat offenders, and you can be infected with gonorrhea or chlamydia more than once.

About 19 million new STIs are estimated to occur each year. Almost half of new infections are among young people ages fifteen to twenty-four.

**Testing**   Testing can be done with a swab of the cervix or urethra, or with a urine sample.

**Treatment**   Both infections are treated with antibiotics. But if left untreated, either can lead to a pelvic inflammatory disease, chronic pelvic pain, and infertility. Alert! Your partner(s) will need treatment, too.

## Herpes

Your initial herpes outbreak—which usually happens within a few weeks after being exposed to the infection—is likely to be your worst. So don't freak out; later attacks are likely to be less severe. The first time you might have painful blisters, fever, headache, joint pain, flu symptoms, enlarged lymph nodes, and a tough time peeing. Sores can be in the vagina, vulva, buttocks, butt, thighs, and mouth. As if that's not enough, new lesions can keep appearing for five to seven days. But after two or three weeks, you'll be clear of symptoms. It might feel like an eternity. It's not. But it's also not over for an eternity. You can experience recurrent outbreaks especially with common triggers like stress, sunlight, menstruation, fatigue, or getting sick.

*If you love something, set it free. Just don't be surprised if it comes back with herpes...*
*—Chuck Palahniuk*

A lot of women get a warning sign and have symptoms such as tingling or itching before blisters develop. But keep this in mind: You might have an active herpes outbreak in your body but nothing to show for it. That's good for you—but bad for your partner if you're having sex. The virus can be transmitted even without symptoms during vaginal, anal, or oral sex. Exposure to a cold sore during oral sex could also spread the disease.

**Testing**   Diagnosis can be confirmed with a culture or blood test, but results may be confusing and need to be interpreted individually.

**Treatment**   Includes antiviral medication, oral pain-killers, topical analgesics, and comfort measures such as baths, good hygiene, and avoidance of tight clothing. Keep in mind that although herpes is a lifelong condition that cannot be cured, the infection can be managed.

## HPV

The HPV virus causes genital warts and, worse, most cervical cancer cases. It's spread by skin-to-skin contact including sexual intercourse, oral and anal sex, and hand-to-genital contact. But you're unlikely to become infected by touching inanimate objects. Unfortunately, condoms provide only partial protection from HPV, since they won't cover all exposed genital skin. HPV is tenacious. It may persist even if you don't have symptoms, and once is often not enough. You can get it again. If you discover skin-colored or pink growths, which look like tiny pieces of cauliflower on your labia, or around your anus, it might be an HPV wart. You may not see any and you may not feel any, but they can still be there. Typically these warts won't cause pain or itching. Even though the warts themselves aren't dangerous, they can freak us out. Get this: Warts can occur weeks, to a year, after exposure to HPV.

**Testing**   Diagnosis is usually made with exam and application of a dilute acetic acid (vinegar-like) solution. A biopsy will confirm it.

### HPV Prevention—The Vaccine

The vaccine can prevent HPV—and ultimately cervical cancer. The shot is best given to women before their sexual "debut." That probably leaves a lot of us out. HPV infection can cause an abnormal Pap smear and, if persistent, can cause cervical precancer and down the road—cancer. It takes at least twenty years for HPV infection to cause cervical cancer, which is more common in women with lots of sex partners, with a smoking habit, and with a weak immune system. See "Pap Smear, Papilloma Virus, and Protection for All Lovely Lady Flowers" (page 126) for more information on the HPV vaccine.

**Treatment**   There are several medicines that can treat warts; in severe cases, freezing, surgery, or laser removal is used.

### Trichomonas

Be careful what you touch! Unlike the other STIs, this infection can live on inanimate objects, including vibrators. Women can also catch it from other women or men. Symptoms include a foul-smelling discharge with burning and itching, urinary frequency, painful sex, and bleeding after intercourse.

**Testing**   Diagnosis is made with a physical exam and evaluation of vaginal secretions.

**Treatment**   Involves oral antibiotics and avoiding intercourse for at least a week after partners are treated.

### Pubic Lice or Crabs

You usually pick up lice or crabs through sexual contact, but the minuscule buggers aren't fussy. They'll travel on clothing, bedsheets, or towels. The pubic louse is a small, round, wingless insect that lays eggs in pubic hair. You'll know you've got them because they'll make you itch like crazy.

A patient with crabs came to see me complaining that her dog had given her fleas. "Tiny black bugs are crawling all over my pubes!" I had to break the news: It's not Fido's fault.

**Testing**   Diagnosis is made with visual inspection for lice or crabs, which look like small black spots that move.

**Treatment**   Medicated lotion or shampoo is recommended, and all partners should be treated. Clothing, towels, and bedding used within three days prior to treatment should be washed in hot water and dried in a hot dryer or cleaned at the dry cleaners. Items that can't be washed or dry cleaned should be placed in a sealed plastic bag for two weeks.

## Syphilis

This STD is an ancient ailment, but it's still a happening story. Syphilis can occur in different stages. The initial symptom is a called a chancre (an ulcerated nontender genital or oral sore). If untreated, it's followed by a rash on the hands and feet, and then neurologic and cardiac issues—among other possible problems. Flash alert! In some cases, there are *no* symptoms. Those at high risk for syphilis have a history of multiple sexual partners. Syphilis can be passed to an unborn fetus from an infected mother through the placenta. Get tested.

**Testing**   A blood test will diagnose the disease.

**Treatment**   If a test is positive, antibiotics can cure the early stage of the disease.

## Hepatitis

You might know the adage: *Love your liver. Live longer.* Unfortunately, hepatitis targets the liver. Types B and C can spread person-to-person when bodily fluids are exchanged during sex; infected needles are used for tattooing, acupuncture, or piercings; or toothbrushes, razors, or drug needles are shared with an infected person. Hepatitis B and C can be passed from a pregnant mom to her unborn child. The good news is that it's still safe to kiss, share eating utensils, breast-feed, and sneeze or cough around others. At first, hepatitis B causes flulike symptoms. Some infected people get yellowing of the skin and eyes (jaundice). One in twenty sufferers will end up with a chronic infection and more serious liver damage. Hepatitis C often causes subtle, or even no, symptoms.

Note: The Hepatitis A virus is carried in the stool of infected people and is usually spread through food when an infected person does not wash her or his hands after using the bathroom and then touches food, a surface, or another person's mouth. It's not considered an STI.

**Testing**   Blood testing is diagnostic.

**Treatment**   Includes medicines that fight the virus.

### HIV (Human Immunodeficiency Virus)

HIV is not an instant death sentence. Yes, it affects the body's immune system, and those with the disease have trouble fighting off infections and cancer, but there are drugs that can help keep it at bay. Still, it's not something you want to get. You can become infected if blood or body fluid, like semen, enters your body. HIV can be transmitted during pregnancy, birth, and breast-feeding. (Medication can reduce this risk.) Early symptoms of HIV infection include flulike symptoms, enlarged lymph nodes, and rash. Infections involving the lungs, brain, eyes, and mouth can occur later. AIDS (Acquired Immunodeficiency Syndrome) is the end stage of HIV infection.

**Testing**   Diagnosis is made with blood or saliva testing.

**Treatment**   Includes antiviral medications and medication to prevent or treat resulting infections.

# I've Been with Someone Who Has an STI and We Had Sex. Is There Anything I Can Do—*Now?*

See your doctor for testing and postexposure treatment or vaccination. *Try* not to freak out! In many cases, the risk of infection is low.

## The Best Ways to Prevent STIs

In a nutshell: Practice *safe sex*! Get tested! Use condoms! Get immunized! Be educated! And review these helpful tips:

- Use latex condoms. They reduce the risk of STIs. Natural membrane condoms may not. However, avoid latex if you are allergic. (Spermicidal condoms may increase the risk of urinary tract infections or symptoms of irritation in some women.)
- Use a new condom from beginning to end with each act of intercourse.
- Use the female condom, which is available OTC and protects from STIs. However, it's not commonly used because it's a drag. It's cumbersome, noisy during sex, and expensive. It should *not* be used in combination with a male condom or during anal sex.
- Use water-based lubricants such as K-Y Jelly, Astroglide, saliva, or glycerin. Do *not* use oil-based lubricants such as baby oil, cold creams, edible oils, whipped

Male circumcision, which removes the skin that covers the tip of the penis, is typically done in the first ten days of life. It may be associated with lower rates of STIs, specifically HIV and HPV infections, and cervical cancer in the women they have sex with. We're just sayin'...

cream, hand and body lotions, rubbing alcohol, suntan oil, mineral oil, or petroleum jelly with latex condoms.

- Consider preventative vaccinations, which are available to prevent HPV and hepatitis A and B.
- Take prophylactic medications, those designed and used to prevent a disease from occurring, which include suppressive medication for herpes, postexposure immunoglobulin injection for hepatitis B, postexposure medication for HIV, and immediate treatment after sexual assault.
- Modify behavior that leads to unsafe situations. For example, alcohol or drug use can lead to risky behavior. Also, multiple sex partners and anonymous partners who met online, for example, are associated with an increased risk of STIs.
- Let your partner know if you're infected to prevent the spread of STIs and help treatment efforts.

# T

# Toys, Toys, and More Toys

*Carrie:* I'm not going to replace a man with some battery-operated device.

*Miranda:* You haven't met "The Rabbit."

*Samantha:* Oh come on, if you're going to get a vibrator, at least get one called "The Horse."

—Sex in the City

Hello, women, Robin here. As a former sex advice columnist it seems entirely appropriate I write about toys! toys! toys! So, this chapter is mine ... and well, yours too. Dr. D. chimes in with important medical and safety info, too, so you get the whole hot picture. Have fun!

Cock rings, vibrators, fluffy handcuffs, fanciful whips, nipple clamps, French ticklers, vibrators, dildos, and penis rings—let me tell you, hot sisters, there's a plethora of sex toys out there, and we're using them. Plenty of women happily share steamy tales of battery-operated multiple orgasms. On the other hand, sex toys can be, how shall we say this? *A touchy subject* for partners who may be under the silly impression that if a woman pulls out a vibrating penis with rabbit ears, she's somehow giving the impression that his penis is less than impressive. Well, as those women who adore the use of their toys report, nothing could be farther from the electrifying truth. Sex toys only enhance the experience. And besides, toys aren't *just* for sticking in orifices. As every girlfriend with a pulse knows, nothing compares with the loving touch of our partner. So let's explore the merchandise in the toy shop and discuss the many ways to play.

In a recent *Redbook* magazine survey of 100,000 married women, 39 percent reported using vibrators during sex, and 11 percent enjoyed theirs to be penis-shaped. Unsurprisingly, 97 percent of these women found sex toys to be superpleasurable.

## I'm Interested in Buying a Sex Toy, But to Tell the Truth I Don't Know the Difference between a Dildo and a Vibrator. How Do I Know Which Way to Go?

Let me tell you. Basically, vibrators are battery-operated or electrically powered (not recommended) devices that buzz or vibe. These nifty items are used mainly for external stimulation. So, if you're looking for clitoral titillation (which most of us need to climax), a vibrator is your best option. There are several different types you can try:

- Egg or Bullet—has a speed control lever and can be used for solo satisfaction or with your partner. It can easily fit between the two of you.
- Hand-free model—is held in place with straps that look like a panty.

- Simple body massager—you can use these on either your clit or sore muscles. FYI: These are pretty powerful items and are often recommended for women trying to achieve an orgasm for the first time. *Bring out the big guns!*

A dildo is an excellent choice if you want the feeling of penetration. It looks like a penis, usually doesn't vibrate, and can be put in your vagina or used anally. (If you're into backdoor play, make sure the dildo has a base specifically designed for this entry so it doesn't slide up where it's no longer welcome!) Dildos can be freestanding or strapped on with a harness. Strap-ons are made in a wide variety of styles, with variations in how the harness fits the wearer and how the dildo attaches to the harness. Often they come with special features to bump up stimulation of the wearer and her sexual partner. When you choose a dildo, think about the length and width you want. (If only life were that easy.) And if you're looking for G spot stimulation, opt for a phallic-shaped toy with a specially curved top. For the best of all worlds, check out the popular Rabbit. It's a two-in-one toy: The swirling shaft offers the pleasure of penetration, while the buzzing "rabbit ears" stimulate your clit.

> Back in the fifties Kinsey days, only 11 percent of the women in the landmark study reported using toys such as vibrators or streams of water while masturbating. Were they too embarrassed to be honest? *What do you think?*

## My Guy Wants to Experiment with His Own Sex Toys. Got Any Ideas?

Sure. One of the best-known and best-loved male sex toys is the penis ring. It's placed around the base of his shaft and constricts blood flow. This may sound torturous to you, but believe me, guys get off on it. Here's why: It increases sensitivity and also promotes a firmer and longer-lasting erection. (And they call this a guy's sex toy?) One type of penis ring is made of soft material, like leather or nylon, that fastens closed. There are also continuous O-rings with no fastener, which can be made of pliable material or metal. But keep in mind, these rings can be tougher to remove and are definitely not for beginners. Another note to beginners: Stay away from metal.

Want to share the pleasure? Choose a soft rubbery ring for him with an attached bullet vibrator for you.

## I'm Tired of My Old Toys and Want to Experiment with New Ones. Can You Suggest Any?

Oh, where to begin? How about here:

**HITACHI VIBRATOR**   This isn't for the fainthearted or those who are new to vibrators. The two-speed, high-powered wand is intensely stimulating and incredibly satisfying, so if you like your toys high powered, then you'll love how hard the motor in this wand works. With its twelve-inch length and two-inch diameter spongy head, the size won't disappoint. The neck of the vibe is firm yet flexible, so you can easily massage those hard-to-reach places! For your ultimate satisfaction, you can set the speed to fast (6,000 rpm) or slow (5,000 rpm), and the electric DC operation in the device allows for constant and long-lasting power. If

Q. The most recorded orgasms for a lucky sister?
A. 134 in an hour
—*Kinsey report*

you're feeling brave, you can buy attachments that'll give maximum pleasure.

**THE BIG O!**  If you're looking for a vibrator with a little more girth, then this is the vibe for you. The Big O! is velvety smooth, firm but bendable, and very long and thick. As with most rabbit vibrators, the Big O! has a rotating shaft, but an additional feature here is that the rabbit ear clitoral stimulator rotates, too, and it's waterproof. The lovely velvety texture means you'll probably do well to have some lube handy. The vibrations are quite buzzy, and there are three different speeds that you may have to take slowly—even when set to the lowest setting, it feels quite powerful.

In 1999, William H. Pryor Jr., an assistant attorney general in Alabama commenting on a case involving sex toys, was quoted as saying there is no "fundamental right for a person to buy a device to produce orgasm." On Valentine's Day, 2007, a federal appeals court upheld Alabama's law prohibiting the sale of sex toys.

**WE-VIBE**  This is one of the best couples' toys on the market. Not only is the We-Vibe well designed and of excellent quality, it's also wire and battery free. The new updated We-Vibe is flexible and easy to clean, and has the advantage of a push on-off switch, which takes you through the seven pulsing and vibrating speeds. The G spot vibrator fits snugly internally with the flexible clitoral stimulator bending around comfortably to stimulate the clit. This vibe works wonders alone, but really comes into its own when used during sex.

**LOVEHONEY SQUEEL**  This is the ultimate toy for oral play. It may not look like it's going to give you the orgasm of the century—it doesn't vibrate and you can't use it internally—but looks can be deceiving, and the proof

## Keep Your Toys Clean and Be Safe

- Read instructions before using.

- Avoid material that could give you an allergic reaction (such as latex).

- Wash your toys with antibacterial soap and hot water before and after use and let them dry completely.

is in the testing. The Lovehoney Squeel has ten rotating synthetic tongues that can be set at three different speeds, low, medium, and high. Even at the lowest setting you'll be amazed at how realistic the rotating tongues are—the Squeel re-creates the experience of oral sex. Just make sure you use plenty of lube, and you'll be pushed to know the difference. Not only is it quiet, but if you position the Squeel carefully, you can go hands free.

**COSMOSUTRA**  If you're new to bondage, then the Cosmosutra soft bondage set really is the perfect way to introduce more excitement into the bedroom. The packaging oozes sensuality and luxury. The ties are all soft, and the ankle and wrist pads are lined with the velvety smooth fabric.

**EVERYDAY ITEMS**  For the truly budget-conscious gal, you can just make use of everyday stuff that you have around the house. You know what they say about *creativity being the mother of blah blah* ... for example:

**Cell Phone**  Put it on vibrate, and it'll give you and your guy's hot spots a body-quivering buzz. Or use the video function to record a sexy flick.

**Bobby Pins**   Use the pointy end to lightly draw circles around, but not quite touching, his nipples. As the circles get closer and closer to his headlights, his anticipation will build, causing them to get erect. Then take it up a notch and use as mini nipple clamps.

**Panties**   Tie your lacy underwear around the base of his penis. The very slight constriction will help him maintain a harder erection, and once he climaxes, the release will be extra intense.

## I Like to Role-Play with My Partner and Use My Toys to Help Move the Story Along—Is That Weird?

Weird? Nah. Wise? Well, of course—as long as you're taking the proper precautions. Whether you're playing maid/servant, boss/employee, master/slave, mad scientist/victim, stripper/customer, doctor/patient, or cop/bad girl, props like handcuffs, whips, nipple clips, dildos, and the like must be handled with special care. You don't want to get into any kind of danger zone—especially when there are foreign objects involved. Make sure you both agree on the same "safe word" that'll automatically stop the action if one of you feels it's going too far. Read the instructions first before using any toy—and follow them. Now go ahead, kids, and have fun.

> Women are getting less and less caught up on an unrealistic and puritanical vision of what a good girl is. When they can embrace their self-stimulation, they can take ownership of their sexuality.
> —Dr. Laura Berman

# U
## Urinary Issues and U

OMG. I'm shopping for shoes when suddenly out of the blue I have to pee like crazy. I sprint out of the store and into the nearest Starbucks bathroom. My pee is burning as if it's boiled water, and I'm not sure if I'm going to die from the agony—or the embarrassment of whimpering out loud.

## What's a Urinary Tract Infection?

Our urinary tract is made up of the kidneys, ureters, bladder, and urethra. A urinary tract infection is simply … an infection. Just like manicures, women are more likely than men to get them. But it's not a cosmetic issue—it's biological. Our urethra is short, and bacteria travel there easily. And the urethra is physically close to the rectum where there are lots of bacteria. Most UTIs involve the bladder (cystitis) or the

How deep is the ocean? Oh, I mean the vagina? Between three and six inches.

urethra (urethritis). The infection usually causes pain, but the good news is that these infections are pretty easy to treat. Occasionally, bacteria may travel from the bladder to the kidneys and cause a more serious infection called pyelonephritis. But let's try not to think about that now.

# Are There Symptoms?

You bet! And chances are if you have a UTI you'll know it—although some women won't experience any symptoms at all. Sometimes your doctor can be sure of the diagnosis just by listening to your description of how it came on and how you're feeling now. Some cases might not be so easy to diagnose.

### Common UTI Symptoms
- Pain or a burning feeling during urination.
- A feeling of urgency, or feeling the need to urinate frequently.
- A change in the appearance of your urine, either bloody (red) or cloudy (containing pus).
- Pain or pressure in the lower pelvis or in the area of the pubic bone.
- Passing only an itty-bitty amount of urine even when your urge to urinate is strong.

### Other Symptoms
- You feel wiped out and weak.
- There's a heaviness in your lower belly to the point of feeling pressure around the area.
- Back or pain on one side of your upper middle back.

Fever is not common if the infection is in the lower urinary tract (urethra or bladder), but it may happen, especially if your infection spreads to the kidneys or blood. Chills, nausea, and vomiting may also occur. Urine may contain blood, which indicates that the infection has already gone far. Don't wait a nanosecond. *These symptoms require immediate medical attention.*

## What Causes a UTI?

UTIs are usually caused by having plenty of sex, otherwise known as too much of a good thing. Bacteria near the vagina can get into the urethra and bladder from contact with the penis, fingers, or devices. As Cyndi Lauper told us, "Girls just wanna have fun," and if that means lots of sex (especially after a dry spell), you'll be more likely to get the infection. It's no wonder the infection is nicknamed "honeymoon cystitis." And get this: Doing the "right" thing by using spermicides, a diaphragm, or a sponge may contribute to more frequent UTIs.

There's a good chance you've already had at least one UTI. One woman in five develops the infection during her lifetime, and lots more have the ailment more than once.

But we can't always blame our UTIs on a shag fest. There are other causes. When the bladder doesn't empty completely, for example, because of a urinary tract stone or a problem with the pelvic muscles or nerves, infections can also happen. Those with diabetes, obesity, and sickle cell disease are at risk. And menopause increases the risk of UTI, since the level of estrogen around the urethra diminishes, causing the tissue to be more delicate. Women with genital prolapse—relaxation of the uterus, bladder, or rectum—are prone to UTI, since incomplete emptying and hygiene may be an issue. UTIs can also occur in pregnancy and are more common if you've had several children.

# How Can I Be *Sure* It's Really a UTI?

Even though you may feel like staying home (or crawling under a rock), you might have to see your doctor. A urine *dipstick* will be used, which is a rapid and inexpensive test to detect infection, but it's not 100 percent sensitive. There's also *urinalysis*, which checks for blood cells and signs of bacteria, and a urine *culture*, which detects and identifies bacteria to diagnose the infection. If bacteria are present, more testing will usually be done to see which antibiotic the bacteria are sensitive to.

If you have a recurrent or tough-to-treat UTI, it's a drag, but your doctor may suggest more intensive testing with CT scan, *cystoscopy* (a small telescope exam to view the inside of the bladder), or IVP (X-ray images of the urinary tract after a special dye is injected into the body).

### Make It a Good Catch!

When you're in the office and the gyno asks for a urine sample:

1. Open the sterile cup without touching the inside.

2. Separate your labia with your fingers.

3. Wipe three times front to back with antiseptic wipes.

4. Let some urine out into the toilet.

5. Catch the rest of the urine in the cup.

6. Close the lid without touching the inside.

# Gawd, I Never Want to Get Another UTI! How Can I Make Sure It Never, Never, Never, *Ever* Happens Again?

Didn't you ever hear there are no guarantees in life? Well, that applies to UTIs, too. But you can certainly cut your chances by:

- Wiping from front to back after peeing or moving your bowels and washing the skin around the anus and genital area well when bathing.
- Avoiding douches and perfumed or fragrant genital sprays or panty liners, and wearing underwear with a cotton crotch.
- Consider drinking unsweetened cranberry juice or taking cranberry pills daily.
- Always urinating before and after sex.
- Drinking lots and lots of water.
- Avoiding the use of spermicides, and a diaphragm or sponge, if you're prone to UTIs.
- Considering using vaginal or vulvar topical estrogen replacement if you're menopausal and UTIs are an issue.

## How Can I Get Rid of a UTI?

Try doing it yourself. There are several OTC products to help prevent or relieve the symptoms. Oral antibiotics that your doctor can prescribe over the phone also work. It's important that you take all the meds even if you're feeling 100 percent at the top of your game. If you stop taking your antibiotics after a day or two, the infection

Make this your mantra: Pee before and after sex—om.

can come back—fast. If you have a really severe infection, then intravenous antibiotics, hospitalization, or urologic intervention may be needed. Let's hope you don't have to go there.

# I'm Leaking ...

You've got urinary incontinence, and even though you feel like the only girlfriend in the world with it, it's a pretty common condition. Why do you think Whoopie feels comfortable doing a television ad about it (besides the $)? There are three different types:

**STRESS INCONTINENCE**   This is leakage of urine because of weak tissues that support the urethra or bladder. Typically, urine leaks with coughing, laughing, sneezing, exercising, running, or walking. This is the most common type in younger women. Your risks are higher if you have any of these: obesity, genetically weak tissue, and multiple vaginal deliveries.

A study by researchers at Worcester Polytechnic Institute shows cranberry juice can change the properties of bacteria in the urinary tract, creating a barrier that prevents the microorganisms from getting close enough to latch on to cells and initiate an infection. Pour another glass!

**URGE INCONTINENCE**   Also called "overactive bladder," urge incontinence happens when the bladder muscles contract too often. Usually, there's a strong and sudden urge to urinate, and before you make it to the bathroom, you've already leaked.

**OVERFLOW INCONTINENCE**   This happens when the bladder doesn't empty fully because it's not active enough, or there's a blockage in your urethra. In this case, small amounts of urine are constantly leaked.

# Why Me?

There are several possible causes:

- UTIs can cause loss of bladder control. The good news? You'll stop leaking once the antibiotic treatment kicks in.
- Certain medications may cause incontinence, including diuretics or water pills, and so can other blood pressure meds.
- Bladder polyps, stones, fistulas (an abnormal connection from the bladder to the vagina), or bladder cancer can make you pee when you don't want to.
- Weakness in the supportive tissues and muscles of the pelvis caused by childbirth, pregnancy, a genetic propensity, and aging can also cause urine leakage. Obesity makes it worse.
- Neuromuscular side effects from diabetes, stroke, or multiple sclerosis can cause incontinence.

# How Can I Be Sure This Is What I Have?

- A good medical history and physical exam will reveal clues.
- A daily log of urinary habits noting diet, liquid intake, and urinating activity, including night-time voiding incidents.
- Urinalysis and culture are standard.
- Urodynamic testing will check the function of your bladder and urethra.
- Ultrasound is often used to rule out pelvic mass and/or residual urine in the bladder after urinating.

### Kick-Ass Kegel Exercises

Kegel exercises tone the muscles around the urethra, vagina, and rectum, which can help with symptoms of incontinence. It make take a few weeks to notice improvements. An extra benefit is better sex!

1. Squeeze the muscles you use to stop urine flow.
2. Hold for ten seconds, then release.
3. Repeat ten to twenty times, three or more times per day.

- Cystoscopy allows the doctor to see the inside of your bladder and urethra to check for growths, blockages, or surface abnormalities.
- A consultation with a urologist (a physician who specializes in care of the urinary tract) is a good idea.

## What Are the Most Common Treatments?

For some, simple lifestyle changes such as wearing an absorbent pad and staying close to a bathroom may be acceptable options. For others, even small amounts and infrequently occurring leaks is just too horrifying, and treatment is sought. It might help to make simple changes that include losing weight if needed, avoiding caffeine and tobacco, moderating fluid intake, urinating on the clock every two hours, and Kegel exercises. Biofeedback may also help. Medications that control bladder activity are helpful for urge incontinence. A pessary, a small vaginal insert, may correct pelvic organ relaxation and control incontinence. Injectable agents can bulk up the tissue around a weak urethra to prevent leakage. Finally, surgical intervention is successful for many with stress incontinence.

# V

## Va-Va-Vooming, Piercing, Dyeing, Vajazzling, and Vattooing

Everyone is free to wear a tattoo or a piercing and I am free to find it ugly.

—*Paul Carvel*

### Vaginal Piercing

Uh, does it surprise you that sticking a needle into the V vicinity may not be everybody's way to go? But if it's yours, the vagina can be pierced in any one (or all) of these areas:

- **Clitoris/clitoris hood.** This is the most popular type of vaginal piercing. Some girlfriends swear it stimulates the sensitive clitoral tissue during sex. Piercing the hood is preferable to piercing the clitoris itself. The clitoris is very sensitive, and piercing it can cause pain and nerve damage.

- **Outer or inner labia.** Only if the tissue of the labia is thick enough to accommodate a piercing.

# I'm Ready to Go for It ... How Does It Work?

First, the skin around the area is cleaned with an antiseptic. Then a twelve- to sixteen-gauge hollow needle with a piece of jewelry attached—usually a barbell or captive bead—is passed through the skin.

Do they hurt? Well, it would seem likely that if you pierce some of the most sensitive tissue in your body, the pain would be excruciating. But get this: Piercing is very quick, and some people who perform and get genital piercings say it doesn't hurt any more than piercing other parts of the body. How quickly vaginal piercings heal depends on the location of the piercing. A labial piercing takes one to four months to heal. The clitoris can heal in one to two months.

Even if you've got the desire and guts to get V-pierced, you might not have the right anatomy. You've got to have a clitoral hood large enough to accommodate a piercing. P.S. You also need to have enough skin in the inner and outer labia if you want to pierce in there.

## Reduce Your Risks

Any time you create an opening in the body, there's a chance of infection. Going to a questionable piercing shop can put you at risk for tetanus, HIV, and hepatitis B and C. Sometimes vaginal piercings can lead to bleeding, scarring, nerve damage, or an allergic reaction. Piercing behind the clitoris may interfere with blood flow.

- Make sure you choose a reputable shop. Look for someone who's a member of the Association of Professional Piercers (APP), which means that the person has at least one year of piercing experience, as well as training in anti-infection and first-aid techniques.

- The person doing the piercing should check your ID, clean the genital area thoroughly with antiseptic, wear gloves, and use a new sterilized needle.

- Choose stainless steel, niobium, or titanium jewelry to prevent an infection or allergic reaction.

- After you get pierced, follow all instructions for keeping the area clean. Wash the area regularly with a diluted saline solution and an antibacterial soap and water.

- Wear loose-fitting clothing to avoid too much friction in the pierced area.

- Don't have sex for at least two weeks after getting pierced. When you do have sex, clean the pierced area with saline solution or clean water afterward.

- Avoid pools and hot tubs until the area has healed.

- It's normal to have some discharge after you get a piercing. But if that discharge is unusually colored (green) or foul smelling, you may have an infection. Leave your jewelry in place, but clean the area with antibacterial soap and warm compresses. Ask your doctor if you need an antibiotic to help the infection clear up more quickly.

> Your body is a temple, but how long can you live in the same house before you redecorate?
> —Anonymous

# Vajazzling

The first time most of us heard the word *vajazzling* was when Jennifer Love Hewitt described it in glorious detail to an incredulous George Lopez. Jennifer said she was "crystalling" her "Precious Lady." Vajazzling is a little like a Girl Scout crafts project. But rather than glue rhinestones onto Popsicle sticks, a professional puts them on your pubic area—more specifically the vulva after it's been freshly shaven or had a full Brazilian wax. (It's safer here because it won't interfere with toilet duties, won't rub off as easily, and it allows for good old-fashioned sex.) This process is no different from using temporary cosmetic adhesive on any other part of your body. Well, okay, it's a little different.

# Vattooing

*Permanent* tattooing of the vulva or labia is very dangerous, and so we can't recommend it—in fact, we won't even discuss it. (Sometimes we can be bitchy!) But *temporary* vattooing is an acceptable alternative. A vattoo starts with a Brazilian wax, clearing the area of any hair and making for a clean palette. The vattoo lasts for seven days, during which you should avoid friction—which means you'll have to think outside the "box." After you've chosen a design from the ones available in a salon or designed your own, the vattoo is airbrushed by hand. FYI: Don't try this at home.

# The Job to Dye for

Did you see the episode of *Sex and the City* when Samantha notices a gray hair on her pubes, decides to dye her mound, and ends up looking like she's grown Bozo the Clown's beard? Well, if you decide to match your rug to the drapes, be careful. You might end up hating the color, and there's also a major chance of irritation on your labia. To play it safe, you could consider Brown Betty. It's a hair dye specifically made for coloring our pubes. It comes in five shades.

Safety Tip: Use a small amount of petroleum jelly to cover the inner skin of your genitals. Be sure to coat all sensitive areas to help prevent potential skin irritation in case any of the hair color accidently spills. Don't apply petroleum jelly on the pubic hairs that you want to dye.

# W

# Waxing, Primping, Smearing, and Shaving

My marriage is going through a rough spot. I don't have time to *wax*!

—*Miranda Hobbes*, Sex and the City

Nothing—nothing—is worse than a full Brazilian wax. Well, maybe childbirth ... MAYBE.

You think you're fashion forward by going for a full Brazilian? Well, think again, girlfriend. Getting rid of unwanted pubes is an old story. Indian women were removing their short and curlies as far back as 4,000 BCE. In Islam, the centuries-old practice is called the act of *Fitrah*. For Western sisters like us, it's still a relatively new trend—and probably the result of our love affair for bare-everything bikinis. Getting hairless may not be a romp on the beach, but these days we get to choose how we want to make it happen.

Get out the grass clippers! The longest recorded pubic hair is twenty-eight inches.

## How to Reduce the Agony Factor

- Stay pale. Don't tan down there for twenty-four hours before and after the procedure to keep your skin from getting irritated.
- Schedule a prime-time appointment. Your body is better able to deal with pain when your hormones are on a steady keel, which would be the week following your period (as if we need to tell you *that*).
- Forgo a foxy outfit. Wear comfortable clothes that won't feel tight and rub against your freshly waxed mound.

# Waxing Ways

Waxing involves using hot or cold wax. If you go to a waxing salon and you're offered a choice, opt for hard (cold) wax. It's gentler and adheres to the pubes, not the skin, which is a big plus. Another choice is speed wax.

Some African tribes enlarge their labia to seven inches in length!

It's soft and sticky and applied with a roller applicator. Although this method is fast and easy, the "ouch" factor is higher because it's more likely to tear your skin. You can also try a natural technique called "sugaring." It's kinder to your skin, but some errant hairs might stick around. Whichever way you go, you'll have to go back again. Waxing lasts only a few weeks.

# Stylin' Your Mound

**AMERICAN**   Some bathing beauties remove only the pubic hair exposed by a swimsuit, so how much goes depends on the style of suit you wear. For a bikini, it would be hair at the top of the thighs and under the navel. This moderate style is also known as a *basic bikini wax* or a *bikini line wax*.

**FRENCH**   Bonjour landing strip! This wax job leaves a vertical strip of pubes in front, two to three finger-widths long just above your vulva. It points the way for his plane to land. French waxing may also be known as a *partial Brazilian wax*. Hair of the butt area and labia can also be taken off. When hair from these areas is removed, it's sometimes called the *Playboy wax* or *G-waxing*.

The Sphinx variety of the Brazilian wax involves the complete removal of all hair in the pelvic region. The name is derived from a naked breed of cat from Canada. The smooth-skinned, hairless Sphinx cat was a genetic oddity discovered in Toronto in 1966.

**BRAZILIAN**   Grit your teeth and get ready to have *all* your hair removed in the pelvic area—front and back. This means hair from the buttocks and area adjacent to the anus, perineum, and vulva also goes. Women who moan at the thought of a total wax-off may choose to have the hair on their labia trimmed. Don't try this at home.

## Yikes! Waxing Can Be Dangerous

You may hate the sight of them, but your pubes are there for a reason. They help regulate body temperature, and catch our natural "scent" (called pheromones) that's produced in our sweat to attract others. Getting a wax literally strips away a layer of protection. It can pull off tiny pieces of the skin's outermost layer, creating a portal where bacteria may enter the body. What's more, the process creates inflammation, which can trap bacteria beneath the skin. Think skin infections (including staph), folliculitis (infection of the hair follicles), and ingrown hairs. It's hair-raising, right?

# Other Ways to Bare It

**DEPILATION**   Depilation uses a chemical to dissolve your pubes, which can then be easily wiped away. Depilatories come in creams, gels, roll-ons, and sprays. On the upside, they're painless and work well, and you can stay bare for up to two weeks. On the downside, some women develop a rash or irritation. It's always a good idea to test the product on a small area first. And many depilatories contain sulfur and stink like rotten eggs. Hold your nose and use in a well-ventilated area.

Rule of Removal: Depilatories should be avoided on inflamed or broken skin.

**SHAVING**   Shaving removes hair to just below the skin's surface, and if you opt for this method, you'll need to do it often. But forget the old wives' tale that shaving makes hair grow back thicker. It's just not true (although it can cause the hair that regrows to be coarser). Shaving tips:

- Nix razor burn and folliculitis: Use a new blade, and shave in the same direction as the hair is growing. Use shaving cream or mild soap, and wash first.
- Avoid ingrown hairs: Exfoliate regularly.
- Get rid of burns or rashes: Use OTC 1 percent hydrocortisone cream twice daily for a few days.

FYI: Shaving can cause skin irritation or razor bumps and may nick the skin and cause infection (folliculitis) around the hair follicle.

**ELECTROLYSIS**   Electrolysis uses a thin needle to zap your hair follicles with an electric current. Hair begins to fall out within the next ten to fourteen days after your electrolysis treatment. It's supposed to be a permanent solution, but for some tenacious types the hair grows back. In fact, there are a lot of downsides: Electrolysis is expensive, can be pretty painful and is time-consuming. Possible side effects include electrical shock, redness, infection, pigment changes, and scarring. As if that's not bad enough, electrolysis could prompt a herpes flare-up.

> Don't try this at home: There are electrical electrolysis devices available for home use that copy (sort of) the devices used by professionals. These machines are often unsafe for use by anyone who's not trained in electrolysis.

**LASER** Princess Leia would love this, since pulsing laser light destroys the pubes. These treatments are safe and effective when they're done by an experienced provider. News flash! Everything has a downside. Laser work requires a repeat performance with multiple treatments and maintenance sessions. It's a good option if you have a lot of hair, but it's expensive. The ideal candidate for laser is light skinned with dark hair. The rest of us won't get the best results. Side effects include irritation, pigment changes, pain, redness, blistering, and scarring. On occasion, hair growth can worsen after laser therapy.

## Compared with My Girlfriends, I Look Like Gorilla Girl. Why Am I So Hairy?

Well, you may have a condition called hirsutism, which is excessive hair growth affecting 5 to 10 percent of reproductive-aged women. Mild cases can be treated with the usual hair removal methods. But if your case is more severe, it might require medical intervention. Speak with your doctor to determine whether you have a medical condition such as PCOS (polycystic ovarian syndrome), CAH (congenital adrenal hyperplasia), or, rarely, an androgen-secreting tumor, causing excessive hair growth. Take it easy; usually, the cause isn't serious and needs treatment only if it bothers you—which it sounds like it does.

# X

## XXX Porn and Lots of Steamy Stuff for Your V's Pleasure

My reaction to porno films is as follows: After the first ten minutes, I want to go home and screw. After the first twenty minutes, I never want to screw again as long as I live.

—*Erica Jong*

Most women I know prefer the UPS delivery guy to bring a package he *doesn't* own to their door. But what can we say? To each her own pleasure: Hard core, soft core. Hetero-Lesbian-Bi. Do you prefer twosomes? Threesomes? Perhaps the gang's all here. Top? Bottom? Vanilla or extreme bondage? There's light spanking, serious "discipline," latex-loving, award-winning role playing, or just playing for laughs. Don't forget (how could we?) cybersex; webcam sex; phone sex; sexting …

# I Love, Love, Love, to Watch Porn. It Gets Me Hot Fast and I O Big Time. But My Boyfriend Says I'm Weird and That It's a Guy Thing. Am I Weird?

Your partner is probably right about a lot of things, but my dear porn princess, he's so wrong about this. Because…

One in three visitors to pornographic websites is a woman!

In fact, according to statistics, a total of 13 percent of women admit to accessing pornography at work. Some search terms are divided evenly among both guys and gals, like the word *sex*. But women and men differ on other searches. For instance, men performed 97 percent of the searches for "free porn." Go figure.

Want more evidence to share with your doubting darling? In a 2006 study at McGill University, researchers monitored genital temperature changes to measure sexual arousal and found that, when shown porn clips, men and women alike began displaying arousal within thirty seconds. Guys reached their peak in about eleven minutes and women climaxed in about twelve. Uh, we're talking like a one-minute diff? Don't be anal—that's statistically negligible.

While the economy was in freefall, a female accountant at the SEC (Security and Exchange Commission) tried to access online porn from her office laptop nearly 1,800 times in two weeks. She also had 600 sexually explicit images saved on her hard drive.

Sisters, it also seems, are more sexually fluid when it comes to viewing the "dirty." When researchers showed gay, lesbian, and straight porn to heterosexual and homosexual women and men, they found that while the guys got hotter faster and more intensely when the porn mirrored their particular sexual orientation, women liked it *all*. Or, at least our bods did.

## I've Read about Getting Addicted to Porn. Could That Happen to Me?

Yes, and it's not a pretty *site*. Approximately 17 percent of women describe themselves as addicted to online porn. According to some estimates, one in three porn addicts is female. Sound crazy? Well, not really. It's easy to get hooked. Here's how it goes: Orgasm releases a dopamine-oxytocin high that's been compared to a heroin hit. Regular

> Everybody got it wrong. I said I was into porn again, not born again.
> —*Billy Idol*

users of Internet porn report experiencing an almost trancelike effect that not only makes them feel oblivious to the outside world but also gives them a real sense of power that they might not get outside the virtual world. The PC becomes their erogenous zone, and the more they try to keep porn out of their mind, the more it pops back in. Eventually the brain learns that porn is the *only* way to cope with anxiety. The only diff between men and women is that we feel guiltier. How *not* surprised are you at that fact?

## We Don't Use Porn to Get Off—I Like to Role-Play Instead. Is There Anything Wrong with That?

Hey, what's with all this "wrong" business? Fantasy sexual role-play can take you deeper into another character and

# Role-Playing Tips from Robin's Sex Advice Files

**Spend Some Time Thinking about It before Putting Your Play into Action:** Some people start out a bit shy and nervous with the idea of dressing up as someone else and playing a role. The best way to get comfortable with sexual role-playing is to get prepared.

**Ask Yourself These Questions:** Who do you want to be? What's the scenario? How can you dress it up? What's your motivation? What (and where) are the boundaries and the ground rules?

**Discover a Fantasy Role That Resonates:** Nurse, policewoman, teenage slut, bored housewife, or dominatrix. Find a fantasy that connects with your deepest self.

**It's All in the Details:** When you first imagine a sexual scene, the main points may be enough to get you going, but the more detail you can add to the fantasy, the more alive it becomes. Details can also be great for awkward moments when you don't know what to do next.

**Choose Costumes and Props:** As adults we don't get to play nearly enough, and fantasy sexual role-play is a perfect opportunity to dress up and have fun. Once you've decided who you want to be, think about ways to add to your character and role through clothing and props.

**Find Your Motivation:** Now that you know who you are, where you are, and what you're wearing, it's time to consider the psychology of your role. Analyze your character. What's your motivation? What turns you on, what turn you off, what pushes your buttons or drives you wild? Are you dominant? Submissive? Do you switch back and forth?

**Keep Those Boundaries:** Obviously, we can't say it enough. Setting ground rules and boundaries with the person or people you're going to be playing out a fantasy sexual role-play with is essential. Some of these rules should be common sense and common courtesy, like no laughing at someone and no judging each other in the moment. Other rules will take some thought and good communication.

**Use Masturbation to Explore the Fantasy:** When we think of fantasy sexual role-playing we usually imagine it involves at least two people. But masturbation offers some of the most fertile ground for developing sexual fantasy scenes. When we're masturbating, we're less likely to censor our thoughts and feelings. Go for it.

release you from the restrictions you put on yourself in your daily life. It means more preparation, and more pretend risks, but the difference is palpable. French maid? Riding ponies? Rubber dolls? Hey, kink is fine, *as long as it's safe*, your partner agrees with the game plan, and your fantasy play time is neither hurting nor affecting anyone else. One rule that may not be broken—EVER: Be sure you have a safe word that will instantly stop the play, no questions asked.

# Y

## Why Your V Skin? Because It's Everywhere!

Beauty, to me, is about being comfortable in your own skin. That, or a kick-ass red lipstick.

—*Gwyneth Paltrow*

## Here's the Scoop on Irritation, Inflammation, Rashes, Allergic Reactions, Ingrown Hairs, and More Misery! Plus the Skinny on Smooth, Supple, Sensual V-Tality.

Don't we have enough to worry about when it comes to our skin? Wrinkles, pores, crow's feet, shrinking lips, sunspots, dry skin, zits, blackheads. Well, you know how it goes. So, you LOL—*not*—when you learn your who-ha can be a hotbed of dermatological disasters. Perhaps "disasters" is too dramatic a word. Let's say simply "unfortunate conditions" and get to the skinny on your V-skin.

**ECZEMA**   You thought you just got eczema on your elbows? Surprise! Eczema is an umbrella diagnosis for lots of conditions that make the skin inflamed or irritated. These include dryness and recurring rashes characterized by one or more of these symptoms: redness, swelling, itching, crusting, flaking, blistering, cracking, oozing, or bleeding. The most common type of eczema on the vajayjay (or anywhere else on your body) is called *atopic dermatitis*. It's often inherited (blame your mother) and a close cousin to other immunologic conditions like asthma or allergies. (You have difficulty breathing; now your pussy is itchy? Not fair.) Affected areas usually look dry, thickened, and scaly. Don't despair: Eczema is not contagious, and there are things that can help.

Even though my patients with eczema see their dermatologist, some feel too uncomfortable pointing out skin problems on their vajayjay—no problem! Your gynecologist can get an eagle's-eye view.
    —Dr. D

**Treatments**   Anti-itch medication, lubricants, steroid creams and lotions; avoiding irritants.

**Prevention**   Try not to sweat (good luck) or stress out (ditto); avoid scratchy materials like wool, harsh soaps, and detergents, as well as other environmental factors that might trigger your allergies.

**LICHEN SCLEROSIS**   This disease is, literally, a real drag. LS is a chronic skin condition that usually affects postmenopausal women. Lose your period, gain lichen sclerosis! It causes the vulvar skin to get thin, whitened, wrinkled, itchy, and painful and most commonly affects the clitoris, labia, and anal areas. Itching like mad is the most common symptom; sometimes it's so intense you can't sleep. Not enough to drive you nuts? Brace yourself: Bruising and cracks or fissures can appear. Even though the exact cause of LS is uncertain, it seems genetic and may come on after trauma, injury, or sexual abuse. LS is not contagious and could be related to other autoimmune conditions. Your doctor will look at it, take your personal history, and then confirm the diagnosis with a skin biopsy.

**Treatment**  Topical steroid ointments are very effective. Occasionally, steroid injections and antidepressants are also helpful. Symptoms may wax and wane over time and intermittent treatment is needed.

Alert! Women with LS of the vulva are at increased risk for developing vulvar cancer. Early diagnosis and effective treatment as well as regular exams lower this risk.

**PSORIASIS**  This is a common inherited chronic condition that looks like red plaques with silvery scales. Psoriasis is not only unsightly but also itchy. For some women, psoriasis shows up on their vulva as well as other areas of the body like their scalp and behind the ears.

Are you scratching? Join the over 7 million Americans who have psoriasis!

**Treatment**  High-potency steroid cream.

**DERMATITIS**  Dermatitis is simply an itchy and irritated rash that you get after you're exposed to an irritant. It could be vaginal douches, deodorants, detergents, sanitary napkins, baby wipes, bubble baths, soaps, underwear elastic, etc. Well, you get the idea. It can look pretty bad, with red, swollen, or weepy vulvar vesicles or pustules.

**Treatment**   Steroid creams and lotions, and anti-itch remedies; avoid known irritants.

**HYDRADENITIS SUPPURATIVA**   A chronic disease lodged in the sweat gland, this condition can infect the groin or anal areas. No one knows why some of us are prone to it, but it's more common in women with acne. Brace yourself: Symptoms include blackheads and red tender abscesses that grow, pop, and leak pus. Tunnels can form under the skin between abscesses, and scarring can occur.

**Treatment**   Includes antibiotics, anti-inflammatory medication, and surgery.

**FOLLICULITIS**   Who hasn't had an ingrown hair after shaving their pubes? Not you? Well don't bother reading any farther, but for the rest of us, folliculitis, inflammation of one or more hair follicles, occurs when hair follicles become infected. Typically you'll have a rash, pimples, or pustules, as well as itching around the hair follicle. It may hurt, too. But it's not just shaving that can cause the condition: There are other reasons like trauma to the skin, obesity, exposure to hot water in a hot tub or pool, tight clothing, excessive perspiration, and skin conditions like acne or dermatitis. Your doctor can make a diagnosis just by looking at it or may opt to take a culture.

Who's happy to have folliculitis? All those hot tub-loving women who thought their bumps were herpes ... and got a diagnosis of hot tub folliculitis instead. That's who!

**Treatment**   Folliculitis often heals on its own, or you can try warm soaks, hydrocortisone cream, or oatmeal lotion, topical or oral antibiotics, or surgical drainage (particularly in the case of a larger boil).

**Prevention**   Avoid tight or chaffing clothing, keep the area clean, shave with an electric razor or a new blade every time (or don't shave altogether), avoid contaminated clothing and towels, and stay out of hot tubs if they're not well maintained.

**MOLLUSCUM CONTAGIOSUM**   Hey, are you going commando in the tanning bed? That's not only bad for your face and the rest of your body (think dry leathery skin, or worse, skin *cancer*)—you're upping your risk for catching the virus molluscum contagiosum. And it's not pretty. Molluscum looks like small, skin-colored dome-shaped lesions with a central "cheesy plug." Ugh, and it's contagious. Even though the skin around it can be red or itchy, the actual lesions won't hurt. Because it's contagious it can be transmitted sexually or by contaminated objects such as towels, clothing, or sex toys—or the tanning bed. And it hangs around. If you don't treat the infection, the average outbreak can last as long as six to nine months.

> It's really time for us to grow up and discover our vaginas!
> —*Lorena Switt*

**Treatment**   Most cases will eventually get better on their own, but options include freezing, curettage, topical silver nitrate, or prescription cream.

**SKIN TAGS**   Skin tags are those small hanging pieces of skin that look like itty-bitty, teensy-weensy flags. They're benign and pretty common. The reason you get them? Well, experts surmise it's just a matter of skin rubbing against skin. So if you're really overweight or have diabetes, you'll have a greater chance of getting one. Look at skin tags as another incentive to watch your weight. Skin tags are harmless and are usually treated for cosmetic reasons.

**Treatment**   Some small skin tags will fall off spontaneously, while others can be removed easily with freezing, cautery (heat that causes thermal damage to destroy or remove tissue), or surgery.

> I've had patients tie a piece of thread or thin string at the base of a skin tag and leave it there to strangle the skin tag until it falls off. It's a crazy home remedy—but it works and it's not dangerous.
> —Dr. D.

**VULVAR PIGMENTATION**   Yes, you *can* go from light meat to dark meat. Increased color (hyperpigmentation) in the vulvar skin may be influenced by hormones. For example, pregnancy can cause hyperpigmentation in the labia majora, tips of the labia minora, and perineum. The V skin can also get darker because of a reaction to drugs or a chronic skin condition. And watch out for repeat depilation or aggressive waxing—both can result in hyperpigmentation if your vag is prone to it.

**VULVAR ACANTHOSIS NIGRICANS**   This skin disorder appears as velvety, light-brown pigmented skin in the groin (along the underwear line) as well as in the armpits, under the breasts, and on the neck. It's been associated with diabetes, obesity, oral contraceptive pills, and endocrine disorders. Your doctor will make a diagnosis by taking your medical history and giving you a physical exam.

**Treatment**   Weight loss, an insulin-reducing diet, and taking care of any underlying condition.

**MOLES** Skin moles can be anywhere on your body—including your vulva—and they can be flesh-colored, red, brown, or black. You may just find one standing alone, or there can be a few in a group. After sun exposure, time in a tanning booth, during teenage years, and during pregnancy, moles can darken. If they're benign (which most are), they don't need any treatment. But moles that are growing, changing in texture, bleeding, itching, or inflamed may need to be biopsied or removed to ensure they're not cancerous.

Q. What did the left labia say to the right labia?

A. If we stick together we won't get screwed.

# The Inside Scoop on Treating Your V with TLC

Glad that's over with! Now let's talk about how you can treat your cha-cha with the kindness and respect it deserves and keep that honey pot moist and lovely.

- Replens is a wonderful nonhormonal daily vaginal moisturizer that lots of women love and use regularly to keep their vajayjay juicy. It's not like a lube (such as Astroglide) that you use during sex. Replens is more like a lotion you might use on your hands every couple of days, but this one goes in your V.

- Some girlfriends enjoy massage (who wouldn't?) with vitamin E oil or even olive oil to help keep their yum-yum elastic.
- There are also vitamin E suppositories that can be ordered from a compounding pharmacy online. These suppositories are in a capsule form and dissolve quickly and easily in the vagina. Hint: We're not talking about vitamin E capsules you get OTC at the corner drugstore; they won't dissolve nearly as well.

> If you have a vagina and an attitude in this town, then that's a lethal combination.
> —*Sharon Stone*

- Some of my patients swear by glycerin suppositories or other OTC nonhormonal preparations (like Vagisil) to help moisturize their beloved V's.

If you want to keep your vulvar skin happy and healthy, you don't want to use chemicals on or near it or cause your V to be rubbed mercilessly. *Down with friction!* Here are some good habits that will keep things smooth.

- For garments touching your vulva, steer clear of perfumed detergents and wash with products free of dyes, enzymes, and fragrances.
- And don't overdo it. Use just half the suggested amount of detergent, no matter what kind it is.
- Stay away from fabric softeners and dryer sheets. *Less is more.*
- Fastidious girlfriends might want to line dry their underwear. (Uh … city chicks: Think twice before choosing this option.)

- Also, air it out. Either sleep commando or wear loose-fitting PJ's or, better yet, a nightgown. Avoid panty hose or be sexy and promote V health at the same time by cutting out the crotch.
- Strip off wet workout clothes and swimsuits immediately.
- And never, ever, ever choose underwear with a synthetic crotch. Let *cotton crotch* be your mantra.

# Z

# Zen Appreciation: Nurturing the Mind-V Connection

*Carrie:* Your vagina is depressed?
*Charlotte:* The mood elevator sort of corrects the imbalance.
*Miranda:* Wait a minute, how do you know your vagina's depressed?
*Charlotte:* There are symptoms!
*Carrie:* Like what, it can't meet its deadline?
*Miranda:* It always wants to go to Krispy Kreme?

—Sex and the City

Kidding aside, absolutely, positively, as sure as Joan Rivers has had nips and tucks, the mind-body connection is for real. If you have any doubt, get this: Research into the science of the orgasm has uncovered that it's totally possible to have orgasms without physical touch or through nonerogenous parts of the body, including the knee and nose.

And it's a common experience to have orgasms through dreams, hinting at the possibility that our mind may be the primary vehicle for orgasms. No one knows for sure why this happens. But just as orgasms produced by masturbation don't differ physiologically from those during intercourse, thinking-induced orgasms appear to *not* be a fundamentally different kind. So, I would say count yourself among the lucky ones if you can use *only* your mind to climax! For the rest of us, a head trip may not always be the boss, but it's so in-charge most of the time.

> It's not uncommon for pregnant patients to tell me they're having orgasms in their sleep without stimulation or recollection of an erotic dream.
> —Dr. D

## Tame Stress

The number one way, maybe the *only* way, to get your mind-set to a sexy place is to get rid of stress and focus on the fun. Really, it's that simple—or not—depending on how stressed-out you are. Sex and stress are linked like a chain fence. Most of us instinctively know this already, and get it when a particularly stressful week zaps us of our sex drive. It's not surprising that studies confirm what we suspect: General stressors in our life can affect our sex drive. That means job stress, financial stress, the stress of being too busy, and especially relationship stress can negatively bum out our libidos.

> Tension is who you think you should be. Relaxation is who you are.
> —Chinese proverb

When we're stressed or anxious, our bodies know it and our vaginas can freak out—everything from losing lubrication or preventing orgasm to getting a yucky skin condition or (gasp!) closing up, otherwise known as vaginismus. May I suggest some proven ways to chill so that you can get hot? Oh, the irony.

# Meditation

Every moment of our waking lives, our minds are busy with lots of perceptions and worries, working on overdrive.

Most of the time, we're not aware of our constant humming thoughts even though they can create negative energy, pollute our physical and emotional lives, and stop our lusty desires. That's because as long as our minds are restless, it's impossible to come into true harmony with ourselves or anyone else.

An Arizona State University study on fifty-eight middle-aged women found that being in a good mood predicted more physical affection and sexual activity with their partner.

Once you make meditation a daily habit, communication with the world will become smooth, gentle, and free from friction. Through meditation you can open yourself to the experience of profound well-being because when you reach the center of peace and quiet within yourself, you simply enjoy *being*.

Surrender comes when you no longer ask, "Why is this happening to me?"
—*Eckhart Tolle*

You're able to maintain an inner balance, purifying your mind and body. Plus, there's a substantial collection of studies to confirm the benefits of meditation for pain management, lowering blood pressure, boosting the immune system, quelling the symptoms of PMS, and of course, bumping up the libido.

## Tips on Meditation

Although meditation has profound effects on our well-being, it doesn't have to be a complicated process.

Advanced meditators may prefer to sit on a cushion in a lotus or half-lotus position and focus on their breathing or on a particular chakra. But for beginners, follow these basic steps:

- Sit in a quiet, comfortable place on a straight-back chair or floor cushion. Relax your muscles; do not lie down.
- Select a syllable, phrase, or word, such as *one*, *peace*, *love*, or *om*, to focus on.
- Close your eyes and follow the rhythm of your breath.
- Repeat your chosen word as you breathe in and out. If your mind wanders, don't quit. Just let your thoughts go and refocus by repeating your chosen word.
- Continue for ten to twenty minutes.
- When you finish, sit quietly for a minute or two— first with eyes closed, then with eyes open.

## Yoga

What? You're one of the three women left in the United States who is NOT doing yoga? Well, just in case you're still in the dark, the practice can free the mind, tighten your butt, stretch your limbs, and keep you a svelte, sexy mama. Here's why: Great sex begins with deep relaxation, which concentrates blood in the central body where it's available to the genitals, instead of being directed to the limbs, which happens when (here we go again) people feel stressed. As deep

Yoga Position for Groovy O's: Upavista Konasana, or wide-legged straddle pose, increases blood flow to the pelvis.

relaxation becomes sexual arousal, the arteries that carry blood into the genitals open, and extra blood flows into the penis and vaginal wall. In men, this extra blood produces erection, in women, vaginal lubrication and increased clitoral sensitivity.

## Breathing

Great sex can be as natural as, well, breathing. That's because breath is the ultimate enhancer of sexual pleasure. It's the bridge between mind and body, and focusing on it can anchor us to the present. It unhooks us from all those thoughts coursing through our brains and connects us with our essential life energy (prana, chi, ki). Breathing creates receptivity in our body and an intimate connection with our partner.

Indian researchers assessed anxiety in fifty medical students, who then began practicing yoga. Their anxiety levels plummeted. Other studies show that yoga reduces levels of the stress hormone, cortisol, elevates mood, and can even improve ejaculatory control. Pssst ... tell your guy to do the elementary yoga position Downward Dog!

Breath control is a multipurpose tool, and it's available to all of us. Shallow breathing allows for shallow emotions; deep breathing can bring incredible emotional release. Each of our emotional states corresponds with a unique breath signature, and with intentional breath control we can actually induce a specific emotional experience—like sexual attraction and superdesire. Alter your breath and you'll alter the experience. Rapid breathing can increase arousal; slow, deep breathing can keep you on the edge of sexual pleasure; long, slow exhalations can boost your sexy self-confidence.

My beautiful vagina is very offended. I'm not offended—my vagina is offended.
    —*Lady Gaga*

### Breathing with Your Partner

- Sit face-to-face.
- Maintain a soft gaze with your eyes for several minutes.
- Next, shift your gaze to the rise and fall of your partner's abdomen and chest during breathing. Place a hand on your partner's abdomen and feel the expansion. By now you may have naturally synchronized your breathing.
- Close your eyes and listen to the breath as it enters and leaves your bodies. Now add a sound with your exhale.

Did you notice a relaxation in your body posture? Did a smile creep across your face? Synchronized breathing is an intimate bond. You are telling your partner, "I see you and I resonate with you."

FYI: You've just experienced one of the basic Tantric techniques.

## A Few Words about Feng Shui

You can turn your bedroom into a steamy retreat by using the ancient art of feng shui (pronounced "fung shway"). Feng shui is about enhancing the environment or the energy around you. Here are just a few ways you can do it:

- First, remove all clutter so positive energy can flow throughout the room. Clutter blocks the flow of chi. You should also remove anything reminding you of past lovers. Photos, love letters, presents, and gifts, anything that reminds you of the past should be removed. You might want to go as far as getting new bedding and even a new

Sex is not the answer. Sex is the question. "Yes" is the answer.
—Swami X

mattress, especially if you shared the current one with a long-term love who's no longer part of your life.

• According to feng shui guidelines, you should get rid of items associated with loneliness. You should not have just one of an item, not one flower in a vase, or a single photograph, or one painting and definitely not one nightstand. Everything should be arranged in pairs to symbolize a union. Have two candles on a dresser, two paintings on a wall, two end tables, etc. You should also avoid paintings or photos depicting one thing.

> I was on top of Keanu Reeves, he was on his back and I was on my trunk, and I was breathing down his neck for hours and hours. It was ... very erotic.
> —*Hugo Weaving, on filming* The Matrix Reloaded

• Water is prohibited in the bedroom according to feng shui. It clashes with the fire element, the element of passion. Avoid having any water features such as fountains or fish tanks in the bedroom, also avoid any photos, paintings, or sculptures depicting water scenes such as waterfalls, rivers, lakes, or streams. Water in the bedroom can lead to financial loss and loss in a relationship.

# Selected Glossary

**Androgen-secreting tumor**   A tumor, usually in the adrenal gland, that secretes male hormone.

**Anoscopy**   An examination using a small, rigid, tubular instrument called an anoscope (also called an anal speculum). This is inserted a few inches into to the anus in order to evaluate problems of the anus. Anoscopy is used to diagnose hemorrhoids, anal fissures (tears in the lining of the anus), and some cancers.

**Biopsy**   Medical test involving the removal of cells or tissue for examination by a pathologist to determine the presence or extent of a disease.

**C-section**   Short for Caesarean section, a surgical procedure in which a baby is delivered through an abdominal incision.

**Cervical mucus**   Secretions made by the cervix. Changes in cervical mucus are monitored for determining when ovulation occurs. During ovulation, cervical mucus increases in volume and becomes more elastic.

**Cervix**   The opening to the uterus, from the Latin cervix uteri, meaning "neck of the womb."

**Clitoral hood**   Also called preputium clitoridis and clitoral prepuce, a fold of skin that surrounds and protects the clitoral glans.

**Clitoris**   The small erectile female organ located within the anterior junction of the labia minora that develops from the same embryonic mass of tissue as the penis. It is responsive to sexual stimulation.

**Depilation**   Removal of the part of the hair above the surface of the skin. The most common form of depilation is shaving or trimming.

**DES**   Short for diethylstilbestrol, a synthetic nonsteroidal estrogen that was used to prevent miscarriage and other pregnancy complications between 1938 and 1971 in the United States. In 1971, the U.S. Food and Drug Administration issued a warning about the use of DES during pregnancy after a relationship between exposure to this synthetic estrogen and the development of clear cell adenocarcinoma of the vagina and cervix was found in young women whose mothers had taken DES while they were pregnant.

**Douche**   Usually refers to vaginal irrigation, the rinsing of the vagina, but it can also refer to the rinsing of any body cavity.

**Episiotomy**   A surgically planned incision on the perineum and the posterior vaginal wall during the second stage of labor.

**Erogenous**  Producing sexual excitement or libidinal gratification when stimulated.

**Estrogen**  A hormone secreted by the ovaries. Exogenous estrogen is used to treat hot flashes, sudden strong feelings of heat and sweating in women who are experiencing menopause. Some estrogen preparations are also used to treat vaginal dryness, itching, or burning, or to prevent osteoporosis.

**Fibroids**  Noncancerous tumors that develop in the uterus.

**Fissure**  A groove, natural division, deep furrow, elongated cleft, or tear in various parts of the body.

**Follicle**  Develops in one of the two ovaries roughly a week before the midpoint of the menstrual cycle.

**FSH**  Follicle-stimulating hormone, a hormone found in humans and other animals. It is synthesized and secreted by the anterior pituitary gland in the brain. In women, FSH stimulates the production of eggs and the hormone estradiol.

**Gestational diabetes**  Pregnant women who have never had diabetes before but who have high blood sugar (glucose) levels during pregnancy are said to have gestational diabetes.

**Hematoma**  Localized collection of blood outside the blood vessels, usually in liquid form within the tissue. This distinguishes it from an ecchymosis, commonly called a bruise, which is the spread of blood under the skin in a thin layer.

**Herpes**   A sexually transmitted disease (STD) caused by the herpes simplex viruses type 1 (HSV-1) or type 2 (HSV-2). Symptoms include recurrent and painful sores.

**HIV**   Human immunodeficiency virus (HIV) causes acquired immunodeficiency syndrome (AIDS), a condition in humans in which progressive failure of the immune system allows life-threatening opportunistic infections and cancers to thrive. Infection with HIV can occur through contaminated blood, semen, vaginal fluid, pre-ejaculate, or breast milk.

**HPV**   Genital human papillomavirus (HPV) is the most common sexually transmitted infection (STI). There are many HPV types that can infect the genital areas of males and females. These HPV types can also infect the mouth and throat. Most people who become infected with HPV do not even know they have it.

**HRT**   Hormone replacement therapy (HRT) typically consists of estrogen and progestin supplementation in women suffering from symptoms of menopause, such as hot flashes, night sweats, and vaginal dryness.

**Hymen**   A membrane that partially covers the external vaginal opening

**Hysterectomy**   A surgery to remove a woman's uterus or womb with or without removal of the cervix. The cervix may be retained (called a supracervical hysterectomy) in many instances. After a hysterectomy, you no longer have menstrual periods and cannot become pregnant.

**IUD** Small, "T-shaped" device inserted into the uterus to prevent pregnancy.

**Kegel exercises** Named after Dr. Arnold Kegel, consists of contracting and relaxing the muscles that form part of the pelvic floor, which are now sometimes colloquially referred to as the "Kegel muscles."

**Labia** In humans, there are two pairs of labia: The outer labia, or labia majora, are larger and fattier, while the inner labia, or labia minora, are folds of skin often concealed within the outer labia. The labia surround and protect the clitoris and the openings of the vagina and urethra.

**Labioplasty** Labioplasty, often spelled labiaplasty, allows for the reduction or reshaping of overgrown and/or asymmetric inner or outer labia.

**Leucorrhea** Thin, usually clear vaginal discharge in the absence of infection.

**LH** Leuteinizing hormone produced by the anterior pituitary gland in the brain. In females, an acute rise of LH, called the LH surge, triggers ovulation.

**Lichen sclerosis (LS)** A chronic skin condition that causes intense itching. It mostly affects the genital and anal areas.

**Mons pubis** A fat pad which covers the pubic bone and protects it during intercourse.

**Morning-after pill** Type of emergency contraception that helps to prevent pregnancy after unprotected sex.

**Ovarian cysts**  Small fluid-filled sacs that develop in a woman's ovaries. Most cysts are harmless, but some may cause problems such as rupturing, bleeding.

**Ovulation**  The part of the female menstrual cycle when a mature ovarian follicle (part of the ovary) discharges an egg (also known as an ovum, oocyte, or female gamete). It is during this process that the egg travels down the fallopian tube where it may be met by a sperm and become fertilized.

**Pap smear**  A screening test used to screen for cervical (and occasionally vaginal) cancer.

**PCOS**  Polycystic ovarian syndrome, a complex condition in which there is an imbalance of a woman's female sex hormones. This hormone imbalance may cause changes in the menstrual cycle, acne, abnormal hair growth, and infertility.

**Pelvic exam**  A complete physical exam of a woman's pelvic organs by a health professional.

**Pelvic floor**  Refers to the group of muscles that form a sling or hammock across the opening of a woman's pelvis.

**Perimenopause**  Also called menopause transition, the stage of a woman's reproductive life that begins eight to ten years before menopause, when the ovaries gradually begin to produce less estrogen. It usually starts in a woman's forties, but can start in the thirties as well. Perimenopause lasts up until menopause.

**PMDD**  Premenstrual dysphoric disorder, a condition associated with severe emotional and physical problems that are linked closely to the menstrual cycle. Symptoms occur regularly in the second half of the cycle and end when menstruation begins or shortly thereafter.

**PMS**  Premenstrual syndrome (also called premenstrual tension, or PMT), a collection of physical and emotional symptoms related to a woman's menstrual cycle.

**Polyps**  An abnormal growth of tissue projecting from a mucous membrane commonly found in the cervix.

**Progesterone**  A hormone secreted by the empty egg follicle after ovulation has occurred. It is highest during the last phases of the menstrual cycle, after ovulation. Progesterone causes the endometrium to secrete special proteins to prepare it for the implantation of a fertilized egg.

**Sitz baths**  Bath in which a person sits in water up to the hips. It is used to relieve discomfort and pain in the lower part of the body, for example, due to hemorrhoids.

**SSRI**  Selective serotonin re-uptake inhibitors are a class of antidepressants used for the treatment of depression, PMS, and menopausal symptoms. Low serotonin levels is currently seen as one of numerous neurochemical symptoms of depression.

**STI**  Sexually transmitted infection, an illness that has a significant probability of transmission between humans by means of sexual behavior, including vaginal intercourse, oral sex, anal sex, and skin-to-skin contact. While in the past these illnesses have mostly been referred to as sexually transmitted diseases (STDs), in recent years the term STI has been preferred.

**Topical analgesics**  Pain-relieving creams, lotions, rubs, gels, and sprays that you rub on the skin. Doctors often recommend these products in addition to other medications to help temporarily ease pain.

**Transition zone**  Area of the cervix most susceptible to precancerous and cancerous change. Also called the squamo-columnar junction or T-zone, it represents the changeover from one cell type to another.

**TSS**  Toxic shock syndrome, a potentially fatal illness caused by a bacterial toxin. It is characterized by high fever, shock, and multiorgan female. In some cases, it has been linked to tampon use.

**Urethra**  The tube that carries urine from the bladder to outside the body.

**Uterine fibroids**  Benign muscular tumors that grow on the inside, outside, or wall of the uterus. They may be called fibroid tumors, leiomyomas, or myomas. Fibroids are not cancerous.

**UTI**  Urinary tract infection, a bacterial infection that affects any part of the urinary tract.

**Vaginal atrophy**  The thinning and inflammation of the vaginal walls due to a decline in estrogen.

**Vulva**  External female genitals that includes the labia majora, labia minora, the entrance to the vagina, and the clitoris.

**Vulvar acanthosis nigricans**  Symmetric, diffused, velvetlike brown to gray-black vulvar skin lesion.

**Vulvar intraepithelial neoplasia (VIN)**  Abnormal precancerous cells of the vulvar skin.

**Yeast infection**  Yeast is a fungus that normally lives in the vagina in small numbers. A vaginal yeast infection means that too many yeast cells are growing in the vagina.

# Index

Biking, 100
Bikini line wax, 176
Bimanual exams by gynecologist, 77
Bioidentical hormone therapy, 87
Birth control, 51–59; abstinence, 58–59; barrier methods, 52–54; and breast-feeding, 59; hormonal methods, 55–57; myths, 95–96; and perimenopause, 81–82; after pregnancy, 40, 59, 95–96; surgical methods, 57–58; withdrawal, 59, 96
Blackledge, Catherine, 16
Blood-thinning medications, 111
Body image, and libido, 122
Body temperature, monitoring, 58–59, 62
Bondage, 160
Botox, 104
Bowel movements, 142–44
Brazilian waxing, 175, 177
Breast exams, 76
Breast pain, and menopause, 85
Breast-feeding and birth control, 40, 59
Breathing, 199–200

CAH (congenital adrenal hyperplasia), 180
Calcium supplements, 113, 116–17
Calendar method of birth control, 58

Cancer, 127–28; cervical, 131; uterine, 110; vaginal, 135
Candida (yeast infections), 67–68, 101
Cervical cancer, 131
Cervical caps, 54
Cervical cells, 126–27
Cervical mucous, monitoring, 59
Chicago, Judy, 22
Childbirth. See Pregnancy and childbirth
Chlamydia, 147
Circumcision: female, 93; male, 153
Clitoral suction devices, 124
Clitoris, 34, 124
Clondine, and hot flashes, 87
Clothing, 49, 50, 100–101, 193–94
Coitus interruptus (withdrawal) as birth control, 59, 96
Colonoscopy, 142
Colposcopy, 130
Condoms, 54, 153; myths, 97
Cone biopsy, 131
Congenital adrenal hyperplasia (CAH), 180
Constipation, 144
Cosmetic surgery, 102–107
Crabs, 150–51
Cramps, menstrual, 111
Cystoscopy, 165, 169
Cysts: Bartholin's, 132–33; ovarian, 92; sebaceous, 134; vaginal, 134

# Acknowledgments

To my amazing collaborator and writer extraordinaire, Robin Westen, I'm honored each day that you chose me! Thank you to Linda Konner, our literary agent; Kelly Reed, our editor; and Ulysses Press. I thank my mentor, Dr. Kaighn Smith, who believed in me from the start and challenged me to "do it all." To my patients, the privilege is mine. To my favorite gyno gals, Adina, Jodi, and Helene, thank you for keeping me sane. To the nurses at Northern Westchester Hospital for your never-ending V ideas; Rose, you are in charge. To my brother, Stuart, the supreme motivator. To my mom for giving me the gifts of compassion and empathy; to my dad for instilling an undying work ethic and unstoppable drive for success. And to my precious boys, Zane and Jace, for hearing more about the V than they ever planned on.

—*A.D.*

I want to thank the brilliant doctor Alyssa Dweck, a creative, compassionate, positive, and unstoppable force who can buoy any spirit and has the most incredible knowledge of everything vagina. Thanks to Linda Konner, our literary agent; Kelly Reed, our supportive, patient and enthusiastic editor; and to Ulysses Press for believing women need an awesome book about their awesome vaginas. And a huge amount of appreciation to all my closest female friends who let me blab on about the V—Laurel (*who* would I be without you?), Helene, Aileen, Martha, Beth, Suz, Lissa, Elsa, Dede, Nanci, Jo, and Sally—and to my sister, Sandy, who is always there for me in a way only a sister can be; and to Dr. Bebop, proofreader extraordinaire. Special thanks to my son, Gabe, who is and will always be my heart's center. Gratitude for my yoga practice and my teachers, especially Tara Glazier, Elias Lopez, and Diana Whitney, who keep me centered, calm, and thankful for my physical and spiritual body. To the universe for all that is and is still to be revealed. And of course, to Sisterhood which is—*undeniably*—powerful.

—*R. W.*

# About the Authors

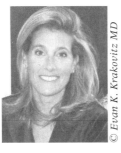

© Evan K. Krakovitz MD

ALYSSA DWECK, MS, MD, FACOG, is a partner and full-time practicing OB/GYN in Westchester County, New York, who provides care to dozens of high-profile patients and women of all ages; she has delivered thousands of babies. A graduate of Barnard College, she has a master's degree in human nutrition from Columbia University and an MD from Hahnemann University in Philadelphia. She is an Assistant Clinical Professor in the Department of Obstetrics, Gynecology, and Reproductive Science at the Mount Sinai School of Medicine and a Consultant (Vincent Memorial Obstetrics and Gynecology Service) at Massachusetts General Hospital. She has served on ethics, quality assurance, and peer review committees. Dr. Dweck is on the Health Advisory Board of *Family Circle* magazine, contributed regularly to *YM* magazine, is a medical consultant for www.stepup-speakout.org, and currently lectures at various Westchester public schools on sex education. She was a research assistant for Dr. Joyce Brothers. Dr. Dweck is an accomplished triathlete who also enjoys sports cars and English bulldogs. She lives in Chappaqua, New York, with her husband and their two sons.

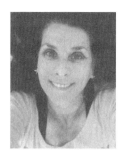 ROBIN WESTEN is an Emmy Award–winning writer and author of several books including *Oprah Winfrey: I Don't Believe in Failure, Ten Days to Detox: How to Look and Feel a Decade Younger*, and *Relationship Repair*, among others. She was the sex advice columnist for *Woman's Own*, a pop-psychology quiz columnist for *Woman's World* and has written hundreds of articles for national magazines including *Glamour, MORE, Family Circle, Cosmopolitan*, and *Parents*. Presently, she is the medical reporter for ThirdAge.com.